Medical Students,
Medical Schools
and Society
During Five Eras

Medical Students, Medical Schools and Society During Five Eras:

Factors Affecting the Career Choices of Physicians 1958-1976

Daniel H. Funkenstein M.D.
Professor of Psychiatry, Emeritus
Harvard Medical School
Consultant to the Dean of the Faculty of Medicine
  on Admissions
Associate Chief of Staff for Education, Brockton
  Veterans Administration Hospital

Foreword by

Robert H. Ebert M.D.
Former Dean Harvard Medical School
President, Milbank Memorial Foundation

This work was supported by a grant from the Robert Wood Johnson Foundation. Editorial assistance was provided by Joan Rafter Ryan.

Ballinger Publishing Company • Cambridge, Massachusetts
A Subsidiary of J.B. Lippincott Company

This book is printed on recycled paper.

International Standard Book Number: 0-88410-704-3

Library of Congress Catalog Card Number: 77-19063

Printed in the United States of America

Library of Congress Cataloging in Publication Data

Funkenstein, Daniel H.
  Medical students, medical schools, and society during five eras.

  Bibliography: p.
  1. Medical students—United States—Longitudinal studies. 2. Physicians—United States—Longitudinal studies. 3. Medicine—Specialties and specialists—United States—Longitudinal studies. 4. Medical education—United States. I. Title. [DNLM: 1. Decision making. 2. Socioeconomic factors—History—United States. 3. Health occupations—History—United States. W21 F982m]
  R745.F86   610'.23   77-19063
  ISBN 0-88410-704-3

To
Henry Meadow
and
Hannah H. Funkenstein

Contents

List of Figures

List of Tables

Foreword

Dr. Funkenstein's book should be prescribed reading for all those who wish to influence the career choices of medical students, and there are a great many today who wish to do so. Most medical school faculty members, as well as deans and associate deans, have a childlike faith in their ability to influence physicians in training by changing the curriculum and/or modifying the so-called educational environment. So ingrained is this belief that others have adopted it without question, and "others" include members of special interest groups, state legislators, members of the Congress and high-ranking officials in the Department of Health, Education and Welfare. Dr. Funkenstein's careful studies have demonstrated that this particular article of faith, like so many others, may in fact be fallacious and factors other than the curriculum or the medical school environment may be more important in determining career choice.

For over a quarter of a century Dr. Funkenstein has been studying the way in which medical students choose careers. Harvard medical students have been the subjects for the most intensive and prolonged review, but he has not confined his observations to one school so that his conclusions have a general validity for all medical schools and all medical students. Several striking conclusions can be made as the result of these studies. First of all, career choices seem to be related more to the general social atmosphere of the time than to anything that happens educationally either in college or medical school. In other words, the general interests of students seem to change from decade to decade and often quite abruptly. These changes are reflected in the changing interests of students in a choice of careers, and Dr. Funkenstein has demonstrated that there are different eras which can be rather sharply circumscribed so that there may be great differences between classes only one year apart. Perhaps the most dramatic example of this was in the late sixties and early seventies. The social activism of that time was reflected in the interest of medical students entering medical school beginning in 1968. Suddenly there was a far greater awareness on the part of medical students of the inequities in our medical care system and a heightened interest in public health, family medicine, and primary care. This heightened social concern now appears to be waning, and it will be interesting to see how this change will influence career choices.

A second important conclusion is that the interests of students prior to matriculating into medical school have a greater influence on career choice than anything which happens in medical school. Dr. Funkenstein can predict with reasonable accuracy the career choices of medical students based on their aptitude in science and in quantitative subjects as well as their social interests. And, finally, students are realists and compromise in their career choices depending on what is available in the way of graduate training and career opportunities.

What makes this book so valuable is the prospective nature of the studies and the perspective it provides the reader on what factors are most important in deciding the career choices of physicians.

Dr. Funkenstein began his studies in 1948 with no preconceived notions. He did not set out to prove a thesis but rather to observe what really happens. He has documented these observations in this invaluable book, and I sincerely hope that every Congressman will read it before attempting to influence the career choices of medical students by legislating changes in the medical school curriculum.

Robert H. Ebert, M.D.
Former Dean, Harvard Medical School
President, Milbank Memorial Foundation

Acknowledgments

The writer has had a great deal of support from many sources during the nineteen years of the project. The work was supported successively by the Rockefeller Foundation, The National Fund for Medical Education, The Milton Fund of Harvard University, the Commonwealth Fund, and the Robert Wood Johnson Foundation. Most helpful has been Terrance Keenan, both when he was at the Commonwealth Fund and in his current affiliation with the Robert Wood Johnson Foundation. The funds for writing the book were supplied by the latter foundation.

Two deans of the Harvard Medical School, Dr. George P. Berry and Dr. Robert H. Ebert, have given help and guidance. Henry Meadow, Senior dean for Administration, to whom this book is dedicated, was the catalyst who made the work possible over such a long period of time.

Of great help in many aspects of the work were Drs. Perry J. Culver and F. Sargent Cheever, Directors of admissions at Harvard Medical School, and Mrs. Tania B. Friedman, administrative assistant in the Admissions Office. A. Noreen Koller, registrar of the Harvard Medical School, aided in compiling the data; James F. Bayley and Roger G. Blackstock were responsible for the computer work under the direction of Dr. Thomas Marx; and Mrs. Joan Rafter Ryan performed editorial work and typed the manuscript. Additional typing was done by Meredith White and further editorial work was done by Nancy Beers and Arks Smith. Carol Franco was of great help.

Dr. Davis G. Johnson, director of the Division of Student Studies of the Association of American Medical Colleges, supplied information. Dr. Harrison G. Gough, Director of the Institute of Personality Assessment and Research at the University of California, Berkeley, was helpful in discussing the results.

Last, and most important of all, are the many Harvard medical students and Harvard medical alumni and alumnae who spent a great deal of time filling out questionnaires. Medical students in the class of 1973 at the University of Michigan Medical School, as well as students in twelve different medical schools throughout the country, also served as subjects. For them, I am most grateful. The deans' offices at all of these medical schools were most cooperative in administering the questionnaires.

DANIEL H. FUNKENSTEIN, M.D.

Medical Students,
Medical Schools
and Society
During Five Eras

Introduction

This study reports the results of a project that examined the career choices of medical students and physicians from 1958 to 1976. It is a prospective study and is written to give an overview of the results.

The major focus of the study was on the relative importance of various factors on the career choices of medical students and physicians. Emphasis was placed on factors affecting the choice of primary care and/or practice in a medically deprived geographic area. Special studies were made of women medical students and physicians.

The unique feature of the project was that it was a longitudinal study. The data were collected on medical students over a nineteen year period from matriculation to graduation. For the most part, this research was prospective, not retrospective. Only a very small percentage of the collected data were retrospective—in order to obtain more information on the Harvard Medical School classes from 1947 to 1958. With data covering this period, it was possible to identify the changes in the factors that affect the career choices of medical students during different eras. Most important, it was possible to determine the factors that do and do not change over time.

Another unique component of the work was the relationship of the data on students and physicians to the societal changes that took place in medical schools, the profession, and society during the nineteen years of the project. Similar data were collected on students and physicians at various times when these societal factors were different. By studying these factors, conclusions could be drawn concerning the relative importance of societal factors versus other factors in determining career choice.

It has also been possible to study the changes in students during the transitional periods from one societal era to another, thus illuminating the factors that make for smooth and those that make for turbulent change. The societal eras encompassed by these data were: (1) the Specialty Era—1947-1958; (2) the Scientific Era—1959-1968; (3) the Student Activism Era—1969-1970; (4) the Doldrums Era—1971-1974; and (5) the Primary Care and Increasing Governmental Control Era—1975 to the present. The transitional periods were: (1) the Specialty Era to the Scientific Era; (2) the Scientific Era to the Student Activism Era; (3) the Student Activism Era to the Doldrums Era; and (4) the Doldrums Era to the beginning of the Primary Care and Increasing Governmental Control Era.*

APPROACH OF THE STUDY

Our primary concern throughout the study was career choice—whether it was possible to predict the career choices of medical students at graduation and beyond from data collected at admission and matriculation. The career choices of medical students and physicians depend upon a number of complex factors that include personal characteristics, values, lifestyle, sex, the economic feasibility of careers at various periods, and the priority given by both society and the government, which is realized in terms of funding and supportive ideology for different careers. By analyzing these factors, we attempted to determine their relative importance in career choice.

Directly related to the career choice of physicians were the issues of primary care and the geographic location of practice. Our concern was with the characteristics of students and physicians who choose careers in primary care as compared with those who elect other careers. In studying the geographic location of practice, we asked, "What are the characteristics of students who plan to practice in medically deprived areas?" and, "What are the differences between those who plan to practice in slum areas and those who plan to practice in rural areas?"

Finally, a major problem studied was the issue of women physicians and students. Attention was focused on the differences in career choices by women and the factors that influenced them as compared to men.

*The designation and description of these eras were developed by this author in a series of publications.

COLLECTION OF DATA

Data were collected on Harvard medical students and on certain alumni and alumnae of the Harvard Medical School.* These data were obtained on students at matriculation and graduation for most classes from matriculation in 1958 to graduation in 1976 and on some of these classes at the end of the sophomore year. In addition, this study used data collected by the admissions committee on these students when they were applicants. Data were gathered on alumni and alumnae from all the Harvard Medical School classes on which data had been collected at matriculation and graduation. These data, collected in 1974–1975, were from the classes of 1958 through 1972.

A random sample of Harvard Medical School students was taken from admissions and graduation data that were kept on file for the classes from 1947 through 1957. Data were also collected on all women graduated from 1949 to 1959. These were the only retrospective data. This project also collected data at matriculation in 1969 and at graduation in 1973 from one class at the University of Michigan Medical School.

In 1975 data were collected on a National Representative Sample of Medical Students. One group of seniors was studied during the spring of 1975, and another group, consisting of first year students, was studied in fall 1975. The medical schools that were chosen represented a wide geographic spectrum and included both public and private schools. Nine schools participated at graduation. They included a western state school, a midwestern urban state school, a midwestern rural state school, a mid-Atlantic private school, a midwestern private school, a southwestern state school, a southern private school, a southern state school, and a New England private school.

At matriculation during the fall of 1975, these same schools participated, but in addition there were three other schools: an urban eastern state school, a midwestern urban state school, and a mid-Atlantic private school, for a total of twelve schools. The schools studied at graduation contained 1,069 seniors, and 479 or 44.8 percent responded; the schools studied at matriculation contained 1,791 freshmen, and 1,242 or 69.3 percent responded.

These data were collected by examining admission and medical school records that include college and medical school transcripts; scores on college boards; scores on the Medical College Admission Test (MCAT) and grades on all three parts of the national boards;

---

*The data will be deposited in the Francis A. Countway Library of Medicine, where they will be available to qualified investigators.

questionnaires administered at matriculation, before graduation, and at the end of their preclinical sciences; personality tests and measured interest tests—in particular, the Strong Vocational Interest Blank; and interviews with a large sample of the students to obtain in-depth material.

Through the above means, data were collected and analyzed in several major areas. For example, data were gathered on the students' socioeconomic and family background, geographic residence, personality characteristics and measured interests, aptitudes, premedical preparation, academic performance both in college and in medical school, specialty choices, and career orientations. Much of the data focus on choice of careers—whether the student or physician plans to go into group practice or to work alone; to receive a salary or a fee for service; or to be affiliated with a medical school, either full- or part-time. Questions were raised about the students' plans to apportion time among activities such as research, teaching, or patient care, and whether the careers they plan are the ones they prefer. If there was a discrepancy between planned and preferred careers, this was explored further. The students were asked about their attitudes and values concerning medicine, and finally, what influenced their career development. The three questionnaires used in this study are in the Appendix.

Chapter 1

Continuum of Careers

CRITERIA FOR CAREERS

The criteria for careers are based on the skills required by physicians in these careers. On this basis, it was possible to place careers on a continuum. One-half of the career continuum contains the bioscientific careers; the other half, the biosocial careers (see Figure 1-1).

Bioscientific careers include careers in basic sciences, which occupy the extreme left of the continuum, and subspecialty practice. Although traditionally Ph.D. careers, the basic sciences attracted a large number of physicians in the 1960s. Subspecialty practice includes the careers of full-time academicians, part-time academicians, and subspecialty practitioners. These careers demand physicians with scientific educations of a very high order so that their skills can solve their patients' problems. For some careers in this category, such as full-time academic medicine, research skills are also needed. Although facility in interpersonal relations and ability to use knowledge of human behavior would be desirable, they are not obligatory.

Biosocial careers occupy the right side of the continuum and encompass two major careers—biointerpersonal and biobehavioral. Biointerpersonal careers demand great skills in interpersonal relations, a strong service orientation, and an ability to apply science pragmatically to the problems of patients. The general practitioner is the acme of this type of physician. Intellectual and scholarly interests in science or human behavior would be plusses but are not mandatory.

Biobehavioral careers, on the other hand, demand a high degree of

5

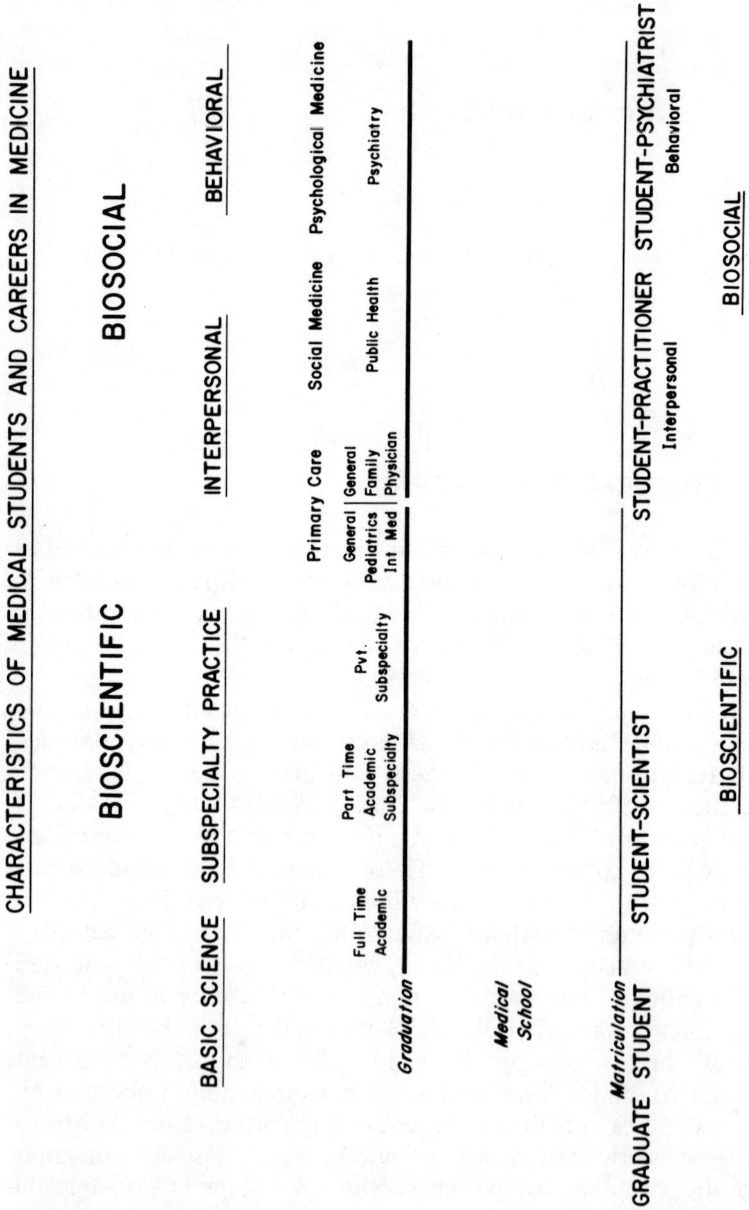
CHARACTERISTICS OF MEDICAL STUDENTS AND CAREERS IN MEDICINE
BIOSCIENTIFIC
BIOSOCIAL
BASIC SCIENCE
SUBSPECIALTY PRACTICE
INTERPERSONAL
BEHAVIORAL
Primary Care
Social Medicine
Psychological Medicine
Full Time Academic
Part Time Academic Subspecialty
Pvt. Subspecialty
General Pediatrics Int Med
General Family Physician
Public Health
Psychiatry
Graduation
Medical School
Matriculation
GRADUATE STUDENT
STUDENT-SCIENTIST
STUDENT-PRACTITIONER
Interpersonal
STUDENT-PSYCHIATRIST
Behavioral
BIOSCIENTIFIC
BIOSOCIAL

Figure 1-1.

knowledge of human behavior and the ability to use this knowledge to help patients. Two careers are placed under this classification: psychiatry and the new public health. In the case of psychiatry, the career is primarily concerned with psychological knowledge, and in the case of new public health, it is most often concerned with the social sciences.

On the continuum, the description of the careers identifies points that represent the epitome of a particular career. Many careers along the continuum combine different degrees of skills and interests in varying combinations. Primary care is the best example of a career combining a variety of skills. For example, the new general family physician needs interpersonal skills, the ability to apply science pragmatically, and an interest in the social and behavioral sciences. As such, these physicians are placed at the midpoint of the continuum.

FACTORS IN DETERMINING
CAREER CHOICE

In this study we found a number of factors that are important in determining the ultimate career choice of physicians. These factors are divided into two main groups—intrinsic factors and extrinsic factors.

Intrinsic Factors—Within The Students

Intrinsic factors include (1) the basic characteristics at matriculation in medical school, (2) values, and (3) lifestyle.

Basic Characteristics. Basic characteristics at matriculation are the students' aptitudes as measured by the MCAT; their preparation as measured by courses, grades, college major, research experience, and so on; and their interests as measured by the Strong Vocational Interest Blank and certain questionnaire items.

On the basis of these results, the students were placed on the continuum. Bioscientific students range (left to right) from the extreme of the student who is a basic scientist to the scientist with some interest in working with people. Biosocial students range (left to right) from the interpersonal student primarily interested in working directly with people and being of service to them to the student with social science and psychological interests and abilities. See Figure 1-1. Many biosocial students combine the interpersonal and behavioral interests, there being a positive correlation between them. There was a negative correlation between the bioscientific students and interpersonal interests.

When the characteristics of these students were further broken down, bioscientific students or student-scientists show aptitudes, interests, and preparation consistent with being a scientist. Among the data that distinguish these students from other medical students are very high quantitative and science scores on the MCAT; extensive scientific preparation, particularly in research and in the quantitative aspects of science; and interest in intellectual achievement. They are similar to graduate students in the sciences.

Biosocial students include three major types of students. The first of these are biointerpersonal students or student-practitioners who are primarily interested in working directly with people and in being of service to them. The second are biobehavioral students or student-psychiatrists who are primarily interested in the problems of patients that involve the social and psychological sciences. The third type are students who combine both interpersonal and behavioral characteristics.

The quantitative aptitudes of the first type of biosocial students, the biointerpersonal students or student-practitioners, are not as high as the biobehavioral students. Their interests are in interpersonal relationships, in service, and in using science pragmatically to solve their patients' problems.

The second type, biobehavioral students or student-psychiatrists, show aptitudes and interests similar to psychologists and behavioral scientists. They are primarily interested in human behavior. Among the data that distinguish this group are very high verbal and general information scores on the MCAT in relation to much lower quantitative and science scores. They are often nonscience majors or biology majors who state, after admission, that had they not been going to medical school, they would have been non-science majors. They thought that concentrating in science would be the best way to secure entrance to medical school.

The third type of biosocial student combines interpersonal and behavioral interests, aptitudes, and skills. There is a positive correlation between interpersonal and behavioral interests, and a significant number of biosocial students effectively combine these skills and interests.

Values. The attitudes of students toward certain factors were studied in relation to career choices. These were interpreted as values using Talcott Parsons' definition: "Values are deeply help beliefs which motivate the individual to action." These include prestige and status, financial rewards, social commitment to change in medicine, social responsibility of physicians, attitude toward patients, the individual patient versus a group or public health orientation, scientifically or people-oriented, and competition versus cooperation.

1. *Prestige and status.* The hypothesis was made that the extent to which prestige and status were incorporated into the student's value system was often one of the chief determinants of career choice. It was difficult to determine this by questionnaire or by interviewing medical school applicants or students because of the social desirability of denying such values. Therefore, we designed certain questions in the questionnaire to obtain this information.

One question gave the student the opportunity to check various aspects he or she liked about medicine. One item concerned the status and prestige of the career. On the basis of previous experience, it was demonstrated that the direct approach to determining status and prestige would not work. Two questions were devised to circumvent this: 'What were the alternate careers the student had considered before deciding on medicine?' and, 'What career would the student have followed had he or she not been admitted to medical school?' It was then possible to classify the alternate careers on the basis of prestige and status. For example, a Ph.D. in science carries more prestige and status than elementary school teaching.

2. *Financial rewards.* Closely related to prestige and status are financial considerations. The hypothesis was made that financial rewards could play an important part in career choice. Hence the question of anticipated earnings for medical students and actual income from physicians was included in the questionnaire.

3. *Social commitment to change in medicine.* Commitment to social change and social responsibility were seen as important factors in career choice. The questionnaire contained several questions on these related topics. Included on the checklist of what students liked about medicine was "opportunity to change society." They were also asked, "Do you plan to be politically active on matters of medical care delivery?"

4. *Social responsibility of physicians.* Students were asked to rank the order of importance of the following factors: art of medicine, defined as attention to the emotional and family aspects of medical care; competence; research; and delivery of medical care. During the last three years of the study, preventive medicine was added.

5. *Attitude toward patients.* Another aspect of values covered in the questionnaire dealt with the attitudes (negative, neutral, or positive) of students toward certain types of patients. Examples included the elderly, young people, children, patients with clear-cut physical illnesses, poor people, and so forth.

6. *The individual patient versus a group or public health orienta-*

tion. A number of questions were used to determine whether a student placed greater emphasis on the individual patient, had a group or public health orientation, or demonstrated no preference.

7. *Scientifically or people-oriented.* At the beginning of the study, a distinction was made between student-physicians who saw themselves primarily as scientists using science to diagnose and treat patients and those who saw themselves primarily as working directly with people using science pragmatically. Don Price used this method to distinguish scientists from physicians.[1] Furthermore, this distinction was apparent in the data gathered from the Strong Vocational Interest Blank. A negative correlation was obtained between individuals with a science orientation and students with a people orientation. (These findings were reported elsewhere.)[2] In a questionnaire administered to chairmen of departments in a medical school, this same distinction was found. Basic scientists emphasized that they were socially committed to helping people but through science; clinicians emphasized the pragmatic use of science in helping people.

During the last three years of the project, when a national sample of students was studied, the Strong Test could not be used because of restraints in the time allowed for testing. Instead, a question was asked whether the students considered themselves primarily people-oriented, scientifically oriented, or a combination of both. These results correlated highly with those from the Strong Test on a sample of students.

8. *Competition versus cooperation.* Competition and individual achievement are seen as necessary for a scientist,[3] while cooperation with patients, community, allied health personnel, and so forth is necessary for the delivery of medical care. Unfortunately these values are antithetical. Part of the questionnaire asked the students to grade themselves on a sliding scale of competitiveness versus cooperativeness.

Lifestyle. From previous work on this subject it was apparent that the lifestyle of the physician was important in career choice. The questionnaire asked the reasons for choosing a certain career, the reasons for choosing group practice, the number of hours of work planned, and the amount of money anticipated.

Extrinsic Factors
Equally important in determining career choice of students and physicians are extrinsic factors. These are (1) the medical school experience and (2) societal factors, especially the economic feasibility of various careers.

The **Medical School Experience.** Faculties commonly believe that the medical school experience is the most important variable in determining the career choice of medical students. If a large number of students in a given class enters a specialty, the professors of that specialty conclude that it is because they are outstanding teachers. This concept was examined critically in the project. Subjects were asked which factors most influenced their career choice—the medical school faculty, the intellectual content of the curriculum, the social conditions of the time, and so forth. The effects of changes in the curriculum were also studied.

Societal Factors. The importance of societal factors as an influence on the career choices of medical students can be understood by considering the changes in medical education and the profession since the Flexner Report was issued in 1910. These changes can best be described in terms of the five distinct eras through which medicine has passed (we are currently in a sixth era). During each of these eras, the social responsibility, the expectations of society toward physicians, the assignment of priorities in medicine, and the funding of careers changed. These changes had profound effects on the career choices of graduating physicians and were caused largely because of societal factors over which medical schools and the profession had little or no control. While these eras will be examined in detail in Chapter 3, we will briefly describe some of their basic characteristics.

1. *The General Practice Era: 1910-1939.* Following the Flexner Report, the traditional medical school curriculum of two years of preclinical sciences followed by two years of clinical work became standard. Science in the first two years was directly relevant to clinical medicine. The objective was a generalized medical education that, upon graduation, qualified the new physician for general practice. There were few full-time faculty, and research was a secondary avocation. Although physicians saw many patients without charge, there was little concern about whether the community as a whole was receiving adequate medical care. Most students took a one year rotating internship and went immediately into practice. The social responsibility of the physician was the art of medicine, defined as attention to the social, emotional, and family aspects of illness, pragmatically applying scientific knowledge to the patients' problems. The role model for medical students was the general practitioner.

2. *The Specialty Era: 1940-1958.* By the late thirties, as the result of astute clinical observation at the bedside and in the operating room in combination with some clinical investigation, it had become evident that it was impossible for one physician to be

competent in all areas of medicine. Hence the Specialty Era began, the boards were founded, and the decline of the general practitioner began. In 1940, 70 percent of the physicians in the United States were general practitioners, but by the early sixties, the figure was less than 20 percent. Graduates began to take residencies after internships. The objective of medical education was to graduate highly competent scientific specialists whose careers were in private specialty practice with or without a part-time medical school affiliation. Almost all specialists were generalists who included a large component of primary care in their practice. Funds were not available for large numbers of full-time faculty members to have careers involving research, teaching, and patient care. The social responsibility of the physician was competence in his or her discipline. The role model for medical students was the specialist.

3. *The Scientific Era: 1959–1968.* During the third era, the Scientific Era, science became firmly entrenched. The founding of the National Institute of Health and the National Science Foundation, the launching of Sputnik, and passage of the National Defense Education Act profoundly altered all education. Society, government, foundations, students, and medical schools gave research their highest priority, and vast sums of money became available. The first two years of medical school were largely devoted to the basic sciences, indistinguishable from the curricula taught in universities. Clinical appointments on the faculty went to physicians who were primarily scientists. Teaching hospitals became more and more concerned with complicated and unusual illnesses; they served a national constituency rather than their adjacent communities. The social responsibility of the physician was to be a scientist, to do research, and consequently to spend only about 30 percent of his or her time seeing hospitalized patients. The role model for medical students was the full-time academician and subspecialist.

4. *The Student Activism Era: 1969–1970.* Beginning in 1967 and peaking in 1969, marked changed occurred that can best be described as the Student Activism Era. Medical students became more interested in solving health care problems than in biomedical research; they tried to change the medical schools by political action. The students demanded that medical schools emphasize the delivery of primary care to all segments of the population without regard to finances, consult with the community on policies relating to the delivery of its health care, educate more minority group students, take action on social factors that breed disease and impede health, and develop a new preventive medicine based on the social sciences.

The principal objective of medical education during this era was to graduate students who would choose careers as family physicians or as public health physicians. Medical schools would develop model clinics for delivering medical care and introduce the social sciences into medical education and practice.

Many factors contributed to the philosophy of this era. Among them were the unmet medical needs of society; the civil rights movement, which brought protest into the open; the passage of Medicare and Medicaid; and the disenchantment with science at one end of the political spectrum by those who felt that it had not paid off financailly and at the other end by those who were concerned about the uses to which science was put. Students were in the forefront of this movement. The great majority of faculty and students did not agree on the new social responsibility of physicians, which would be primarily concerned with the delivery of medical care. In these circumstances, students were without role models.

5. *The Doldrums Era: 1971-1974.* By 1971, the Student Activism Era ended and the Doldrums Era began. Although some model clinics had been established by medical schools and social medicine departments were stronger, the basic attitudes of medical school faculty and the profession remained unchanged. Only two of the student demands were implemented: the education of more minority group students and consultation with the community about the delivery of its health care. The failure to implement the other demands was due to two major factors: the basic attitudes of the majority of medical school faculty and of organized medicine, and inadequate funding.

There was little consensus within the medical school community about the direction in which medical schools should move. The decreased funding of research, the dearth of pre- and postdoctoral fellowships, and changes in the attitudes of society and the government toward science confirmed that the Scientific Era was over, but most faculty still looked for its revival. This was best exemplified by the fact that faculty placed increased pressure on admission committees to select students with outstanding scientific backgrounds. Added to these difficulties was inflation, which exacerbated the severe funding problems. Most medical schools remained in a holding pattern, unable to activate innovative projects. Medical education was indeed in the doldrums, and medical students remained without role models.

6. *The Primary Care and Increasing Governmental Control Era: 1975-present.* Since the end of the Student Activism Era in 1972, society and the government have increasingly demanded more primary care physicians and greater numbers of doctors in medically underserviced areas. The rise in importance of the American Acad-

emy of Family Practice and the establishment of the Board of Family Medicine in 1969 reinforced this movement, in which the Robert Wood Johnson Foundation has been a catalyst. The climax of this effort occurred with the passage by Congress of the 1976 Manpower Act. The aim of this legislation is to increase the number of primary care physicians in medically underserviced areas.

In this legislation, primary care is defined as general family medicine, general internal medicine, and general pediatrics. If schools do not insure that a certain percentage of graduates enter primary care, they will not receive their capitation grants. A certain percentage of students who need funds for medical education will be able to enlist in the National Health Service Corps. Three years after graduation, they give one year of service as a primary care physician in a medically deprived area for each year of financial support.

Evidence of increasing governmental control is best seen in the section of the act that mandates that, to secure capitation grants, medical schools accept into their third year American citizens attending foreign medical schools who have passed Part I of their national boards. Further evidence is seen in the federal legislation to insure the quality of care by the Professional Standards Review Organization (PSRO) and in state laws that require physicians to take continuing education courses to retain their licenses.

The primary care movement is not entirely mandated by government; it is also a matter of economics. There is evidence of overcrowding in certain specialties such as surgery and in the medical subspecialty of cardiology and diagnostic radiology. Careers in academic medicine are difficult to pursue because of the lack of funds for research and faculty salaries. The medical schools will soon begin to graduate approximately 15,000 physicians per year. In ten years, 150,000 doctors will be added to the 350,000 now in the United States. The Carnegie Commission reported that this may produce too many physicians and that projected new schools should not be activated.[4]

The demands of society, the governmental action as shown in the passage of the Manpower Act, the advocation of national health insurance by President Carter, and the current societal factors in economic incentives and ideology indicate that the new era of primary care and increasing governmental control has begun.

Chapter 2

Patterns of Career Choice

A fundamental interrelationship exists between the intrinsic and extrinsic factors in the career choices of medical students. The data on the career choices of these students at matriculation and graduation are presented using two methods. First, the basic characteristics of students at matriculation were related to their career choices at graduation for classes at the acme of each era. This shows graphically the type of students admitted and the type of careers chosen by them four years later. The second method illustrates the changes in the type of careers chosen by students both at matriculation and at graduation in the same chronological year. This highlights the effects of societal factors on students at the same period in chronological time, but not in the same class. The pattern of the career choices of students at graduation, as related to their basic characteristics at matriculation, is described for each era.

THE SPECIALTY ERA

The Specialty Era, from 1940 to 1958 (see Figure 2-1), showed a large increase in applicants from 1947 to 1952 due to returning veterans. Later the number of applicants declined rapidly, and it became easy to secure entrance to medical school.

Admissions committees during this era preferred the liberal arts major with a well-rounded education. Two Buck Hill Falls conferences on premedical education[1] and the data from this project indicate that the majority of applicants were biosocially oriented. In

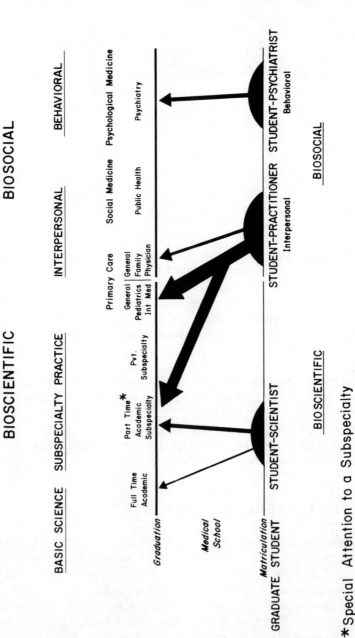

CHARACTERISTICS OF MEDICAL STUDENTS AND CAREERS IN MEDICINE

Figure 2-1.   The Specialty Era—The Fifties

The thicker the line, the larger the number of students.

the class that entered Harvard Medical School in 1958, eighty-six or 75.4 percent were biosocial; only twenty-eight or 24.6 percent were bioscientific. The biosocial group contained fifty-eight or 67.4 percent classified as student-practitioners, twenty-four or 27.9 percent classified as student-psychiatrists, and 4.6 percent classified as a combination of the two.

In their premedical studies, over half of the students were non-science majors with only the minimum science required. Among the science majors, many had followed premedical majors and had studied little beyond the required science courses. Few students had studied calculus or physical chemistry and less than 20 percent had taken one or more social science courses in college.

As far as their values were concerned, students electing careers in private specialty practice saw this career as offering the most prestige, with academic medicine second, and general practice and psychiatry third. The greatest financial rewards were expected by those electing private specialty practice; the least, by those in academic medicine. Few students were committed to social change in medicine. This is demonstrated by the small number in favor of national health insurance (see Table 2-1). The social responsibility of the physician was

Table 2-1. Attitudes and Values Concerning Medicine of Harvard Medical Students at Graduation

	Class of 1959 (%)	Class of 1963 (%)	Class of 1971 (%)	Class of 1976 (%)
1. In favor of group practice	8	6	98	99
2. For abolishing fee for service	4	5	61	56
3. Most important values:				
A. The art of medicine	25	4	7	19
B. Competence of the physician	65	47	35	39
C. Delivery of optimal care to the entire population	0	0	42	22
D. Research	10	49	6	2
E. Preventive medicine*	–	–	–	17
4. Favor national health insurance	9	13	81	76
5. Dissatisfied with delivery of medical care	9	14	86	79
6. Plan to be politically active on matters of health	4	6	68	59

*Not questioned in these years.

seen as competence, with the art of medicine second. Few saw research or the delivery of medical care as a high priority. Positive attitudes were toward the young and those with clear-cut physical illnesses. Negative attitudes were toward the elderly and those with psychological symptoms. Almost all were oriented toward the individual patient; few had a public health orientation. Most were people-oriented, with less than 30 percent scientifically oriented. The students were equally divided between being competitive and cooperative.

It was found in this era that lifestyle influenced career choice. Women were more often limited by lifestyle in choosing careers, often electing salaried positions with fixed hours. Men expected to work long hours. A minority, principally ophthalmologists, chose their specialty in order to limit the number of hours they worked.

The medical school during this era contained relatively few full-time teachers, most of the clinical faculty being on a part-time basis. Moreover, throughout the fifties there were increasing numbers of psychiatrists due to funding by the National Institute of Mental Health (NIMH).

The typical career choice during this era involved the student-practitioner who planned to work directly with people using science pragmatically to solve problems (see Figure 2-1). By graduation, the majority chose a general specialty practice—general medicine, general pediatrics, general surgery—with or without medical school affiliation. Only a few considered a subspecialty.

All of the student-scientists chose careers in academic medicine. The effect of economics on career choice, however, could be seen in that 52.6 percent of the bioscientific students planning part-time academic careers would have preferred full-time academic careers, but lack of funding precluded such a career.

Private specialty practice, with or without an academic affiliation, was economically feasible. Funding by NIMH and the increased acceptability of psychiatry by society made this specialty a more viable career as the era progressed. Many more elected psychiatry in the late fifties than had a decade earlier. In fact, almost all of the student-psychiatrists chose psychiatry.

THE SCIENTIFIC ERA

In the early years of the Scientific Era, from 1959 to 1961, the number of medical school applicants fell due to the low birth rate twenty-one years before and because of the preference of many students to attend graduate school in the sciences. As we pointed out, this was attributable to the great increase in the funding of science following Sputnik and to the corresponding ideology of the time, which placed a high national priority on science. The number of scientists in the medical applicant pool increased rapidly, and by the midsixties there were sizable numbers, although most of those seeking entrance were still biosocial students.

However, the preference of the admissions committee changed from biosocial to bioscientific students. Approximately 50–60 percent of the admitted students were bioscientific. The biosocial students were still predominantly student-practitioners, but now a sizable number were student-psychiatrists. The only constraint to having a great majority of bioscientific students was that most student-scientists preferred graduate school. At the height of this era, 48 percent of the students admitted to medical school were still unsure whether they had made the correct choice in electing medicine rather than the sciences.

Most marked was the dramatic increase in the scientific preparation of all students. The great majority were majors in biology, chemistry, or physics. Many students had advanced standing in science in college, and a large number had taken graduate courses in college. The majority had done research, and the number of biology, chemistry, physics, and mathematics courses studied more than doubled.

Prestige and status shifted in the minds of students from private specialty practice to full-time academic medicine. The financial rewards of those in private specialty practice were still highest, but there was a marked increase in the monetary expectations of those who planned careers in academic medicine. Commitment to change in medicine, which was directed toward improving scientific medicine, increasing research, and expanding academic centers, was great on the part of students, faculty, society, organized medicine, and the federal government. The social responsibility of the physician changed as well. There was a marked downgrading of the art of medicine as research became the most important value. Competence still ranked high (see Table 2-1). Attitudes toward patients changed marginally; the majority still reacted negatively toward the elderly and those with psychological illnesses. Orientation was still toward the individual patient, and there was little evidence of a public health orientation.

There was abundant evidence in the data of the shift away from being primarily people-oriented toward science. This was shown in the changed pattern in the Strong Test.[2] In fact, there was a negative correlation between measured interests in working with people and interest in science. Science was now considered one of the things the students liked best about medicine, whereas during the previous era it was less important. Most students considered themselves highly competitive scientists.

The majority of the students planned the lifestyle of the academician, preparing to work long hours for academic advancement rather than for the demands of patients. Women were still limited by lifestyle. A small percentage of men still chose careers where they could limit their hours in order to follow outside interests.

The accelerating increase in funds for science resulted in a great expansion of research in both the medical school and the university so that their basic science departments were remarkably similar. So similar was science in a university that for many medical students the preclinical years were a repetition of their undergraduate science courses. At Harvard Medical School, the correlation between grades and having had a similar course in college was 0.86. Grades in the first year of medical school reflected the preparation of the students.

There were many new full-time faculty appointments during this era, and the major qualification of full-time clinical professors was their research in the basic sciences. Postdoctoral fellowships were the order of the day, and most physicians in the academic medical center became subspecialists. The academic medical center became increasingly a tertiary care institution, with little attention to primary care in the outpatient department. In fact, at some institutions, one of the chief rewards for being promoted to associate professor was no longer having to work in the outpatient department.

Concomitant with this, funding through NIMH increased for research in psychiatry, for faculty appointments, and for teaching medical students and residents. This made careers in this specialty more feasible. There were no places for general or family practitioners.

While the increase in funding for science and psychiatry made these careers more economically feasible, the downgrading of general practice continued. This was illustrated by the $12,000 yearly stipends given by the government to established general practitioners to abandon their practices for psychiatric residencies, since they were no longer needed as primary care physicians. These were oversubscribed.

Of the 50-60 percent bioscientific students admitted to the school, almost all chose careers in academic medicine, both full and part time, with a slight majority favoring full-time academic medicine at the height of the era (see Figure 2-2). The discrepancy of the previous era between planned and preferred careers disappeared. Those who sought a full-time academic career thought this was possible. The type of bioscientific career changed from general specialty prac-

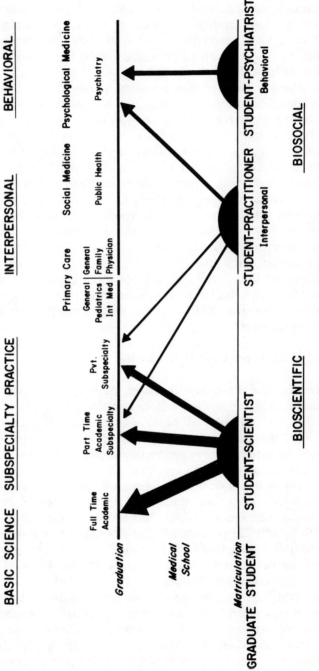

CHARACTERISTICS OF MEDICAL STUDENTS AND CAREERS IN MEDICINE

Figure 2-2. The Scientific Era—1959-1968

The thicker the line, the larger the number of students.

tice to subspecialty practice with a large component of research. Certain schools, such as Harvard, could more quickly capitalize on the new availability of funds, as shown by Sanazaro,[3] who found that a high correlation existed at that time among achieving high MCAT scores, attending certain medical schools, and choosing a career in academic medicine.

Marked changes also occurred in the career choices of biosocial students at graduation. Although almost all student-psychiatrists still chose psychiatry, only a small number of student-practitioners still chose private general specialty practice with a large component of primary care, with or without a medical school affiliation. Most of these students, as well as those combining the traits of the student-practitioner with those of the student-psychiatrist, planned carreers in psychiatry. Some entered medical school planning to become general practitioners, general internists, or pediatricians, but changed to psychiatry because they wanted to work with patients on a close, interpersonal basis. They found the ward and outpatient departments of teaching hospitals "too cold, too scientific, and too impersonal." Many of these students did not have interests in the psychological field, but, being primarily interested in working directly with patients, saw psychiatry as the only specialty left that offered this opportunity.[4]

THE STUDENT ACTIVISM ERA

During the short-lived Student Activism Era, from 1969 to 1970, the number of medical school applicants began to increase markedly, with the number of bioscientific students increasing slightly. In 1969, programs began to admit minority group students, which in turn resulted in increased applications from them. At the same time there was an increase in women applicants.

There was a noticeable change in the preparation of all students. Although they had studied as much science as ever, there were a greater number who had studied social sciences in college. Prior to 1969, only 20 percent of students in the Harvard applicant pool had studied a social science in college; but in one year—1969—this increased to 74 percent and then quickly rose to over 90 percent.

Approximately 50 percent of the students admitted were bioscientific, few of whom any longer struggled with a choice between a Ph.D. and an M.D.; they were committed to medicine. The remaining 50 percent, who were biosocial, included almost all of the increased number of women and minority group students. Another change in this category was that in the previous eras, approximately

80 percent of students showed the distinct characteristics of either the student-practitioner or the student-psychiatrist. At this time, only 50 percent showed these distinct characteristics; the other 50 percent combined the characteristics of the student-practitioner and the student-psychiatrist.

The most marked changes in this era were in student values and attitudes. Prestige and status were downgraded. Although many students had considered highly prestigious careers early in college, such as the law or a Ph.D. in science, when they entered medical school in 1969, they stated that had they not secured entrance to medical school they would have entered social work, politics, or teaching in elementary or secondary schools. They also indicated that they planned to make less money and were committed to social change in medicine. There was a marked increase in the number of students who felt that one of the greatest attractions of medicine was that it offered the opportunity to change society. The students were so committed to social change that a third of them would solve problems by action or by trial and error rather than by careful analyses of the problems before action. The number that would be politically active rose from 6 percent to over half the class. The social responsibility of the physician became primarily the delivery of medical care to the entire population, with the competence of the physician placing second. Research had fallen from 49 percent in the class of 1963 to 6 percent in the class of 1971. In attitudes toward patients, there was also a marked change. This time the students reacted positively to the elderly and to those with psychological problems and negatively to the affluent. The same high positive reaction toward the young and those with clear-cut physical ilnesses continued.

There was strong interest in the preventive aspects of medicine, especially the social factors that cause disease. There was a decrease in the orientation toward science, many now seeing themselves as primarily people-oriented, and a far greater emphasis was placed on cooperation rather than competition. This was best seen in the overwhelming demands on the faculty for a pass-fail rather than a letter grading system.

Significant changes in the lifestyle of students took place. The students planned to practice in groups in order to have more time for their families and other outside activities. The number of hours they planned to work were far fewer than in other eras, and they planned to spend a great deal of time being politically active on health problems. Many planned to work in deprived areas with fewer monetary rewards.

During this era, there was considerable turmoil in the medical schools, because the majority of students and the faculty held vastly disparate views on the role of the medical school. The students wanted the medical school to educate more students to practice primary care in deprived areas and to take action on the social factors in the community that cause illness. Students successfully worked to organize the surrounding community so that they would have a voice in the medical center's policies regarding the delivery of medical care. The faculty, on the other hand, wanted to return to the Scientific Era and to continue its policies. Some model community clinics were established, preventive and social medicine departments were strengthened, more minority group students were admitted, and a pass-fail grading system was adopted (against the judgment of the faculty).

Funding for postdoctoral programs and research grants continued to increase, making academic careers appear viable. Government funding for primary care, however, was only slightly increased. Medicare and Medicaid, which began in 1966, were not yet significant economic incentives for primary care. But when their coverage was broadened in 1973, they did become an economic incentive for primary care. Yet, during the Student Activism Era, primary care was not considered an economically viable career. The Board of Family Medicine was established in 1969, but it was not yet influential on a national scale.

With regard to career choice, the bioscientific group showed a significant decline in choosing full-time academic careers in favor of part-time academic careers, with a moderate increase in choosing private specialty practice (see Figure 2-3). Many of these students planned a general specialty practice rather than a subspecialty practice, the reverse of the choices of their immediate predecessors.

Even more dramatic changes occurred within the biosocial group. In 1966, 55 percent of the students at matriculation and 100 percent at graduation chose psychiatry; in 1969, less than 20 percent at matriculation and 33 percent at graduation still chose psychiatry. In 1969, the percentage of students in this group choosing public health or family medicine at matriculation each exceeded the percentage choosing psychiatry. At graduation in that same year, public health exceeded psychiatry as a career choice, and in 1970 family medicine exceeded psychiatry.

The marked shift in the career choices of these students was related to the activism of the time. The career choices reflected their desire to solve problems of health care delivery and to take action on the social factors that cause disease and impede health. This was especially true in the choice of public health and in the move away

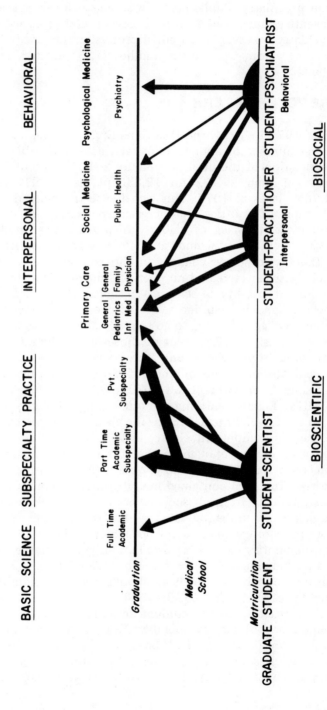

Figure 2–3.   The Student Activism Era—1969–1970
The thicker the line, the larger the number of students.

from psychiatry. Public health was seen as a career that emphasized preventive and social factors in disease and promised social action. Psychiatry was seen as an elitist profession that treated few patients, most of whom were upper middle class, educated, and financially affluent.

THE DOLDRUMS ERA

From 1971 to 1974, the Doldrums Era, there was a marked increase in the number of applicants as well as a noticeable change in the composition of the pool (see Figure 2-4). The number of applicants increased from 29,172 for 12,335 places in 1971 to 42,624 for 14,763 places in 1974. This was due to the marked increase in the birthrate in the fifties, the increasing percentage of students attending college, the lack of viability of science as a career, and the increasing numbers of women and minority group applicants.

There were three changes in the composition of the applicant pool. First, an increased number of student-scientists applied due to the loss of viability of science as a career. This forced many Ph.Ds in science, graduate students in science, and undergraduates who entered college planning to go to graduate school to apply to medical school. In 1972, 27 percent of those taking the MCAT had already graduated from college; only three years before, the figure was 17 percent. Second, the number of women entering medical school increased from 948 in 1969-1970 to 3,275 for the class that entered in 1974. Finally, entering minority group students increased from 501 in 1969-1970 to 1,473 for the class that entered in 1974.[5]

The most important change in the pool of applicants was that it was now diverse enough so that for the first time medical school admission committees could choose almost any type of student they desired. The pool contained many women and minority group members, students from all socioeconomic levels, bioscientific students ranging from undergraduates to Ph.Ds, biosocial students ranging from psychology to social science majors to Ph.Ds in psychology and the humanities, as well as sizable numbers of mathematics, physics, and engineering majors from the baccalaureate to the Ph.D. level. It was now possible for medical school admission committees to decide what types of students to admit.

As a reaction to the student activism of the previous era, many medical school faculty members, especially those in the basic sciences who previously had been unwilling to serve on admission committees, sought appointments to insure that the more scientifically oriented, conservative students would be admitted. The only

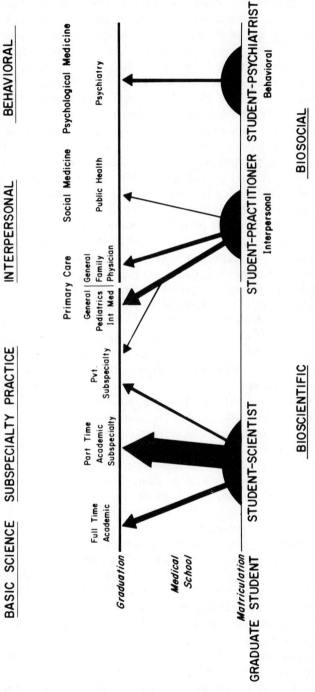

CHARACTERISTICS OF MEDICAL STUDENTS AND CAREERS IN MEDICINE

BIOSCIENTIFIC   BIOSOCIAL

BASIC SCIENCE   SUBSPECIALTY PRACTICE   INTERPERSONAL   BEHAVIORAL

Figure 2-4.   The Doldrums—1971–1974
The thicker the line, the larger the number of students.

factor that prevented the class from being almost entirely bioscientific was the intense pressure on the medical schools to admit women and minority group students, most of whom were biosocial. However, as the era continued and the number of women applying and securing entrance increased, more of them exhibited the characteristics of bioscientific students because many had planned to go to graduate school in science but had changed their plans to become physicians during college due to the decreased funding in science. Toward the end of the era, a small increase in bioscientists began to occur among minority group students as well, since they were now securing entrance to universities that offered high level scientific educations.

Prestige and status were still important values for bioscientific students. But for those going into family medicine or into deprived areas, their alternate career often lacked prestige and status. Financial rewards were still high for the class as a whole except that women and those students who planned to work in deprived areas or to enter primary care expected to earn less money. The commitment to social change in medicine remained high, as evidenced by the large number planning to be politically active, the high percentage in favor of national health insurance, those favoring abolishing fee for service, and those dissatisfied with the delivery of medical care (see Table 2-1). The social responsibility of the physician changed, but not dramatically. Competence was the most important value, delivery of care second, with an increase in the importance of the art of medicine. The state of research continued at a strikingly low 4 percent. During the Scientific Era this had been ranked highest by 49 percent of the students. In attitudes toward patients, the elderly and the worried well were no longer viewed positively by the majority of students, who overwhelmingly preferred young patients and those with clear-cut physical illnesses. A small number, although an increase over the Scientific Era, continued to hold a public health orientation. A majority considered themselves primarily people-oriented, and there was an even split between those considering themselves competitive or cooperative.

With respect to lifestyle, almost all of the students planned to work fewer hours than in the past and to practice in groups to have more time for their families and outside activities. The most striking change was in the lifestyle of women. Although they still planned to practice fewer hours than men, they planned specialties much like men, except for pediatrics. They no longer saw a conflict between rearing a family and having a career. However, there was conflict among them in their views of women's role in medicine. One group felt that women should be primary care physicians or pediatricians, often in deprived areas, because they brought something unique to medicine. Another group felt that women are no different from men professionally and should be in the broad spectrum of the specialties of medicine. These opposing viewpoints were well expressed by three women in a symposium at the Harvard Medical School.[6]

There was a marked generation gap in medical school, both between the students and faculty and between the students and other medical practitioners. The faculty hoped for a revival of the Scientific Era and conducted their affairs as if this would occur. But students saw their career concerns in a much different light than did the faculty. Most medical students did not believe that the medical school played a prime role in their future careers. This was because they had survived tremendous competition to secure entrance; they were aware of the financial difficulties of securing their education and of the financial difficulties of medical schools; and they realized the difficulties many young physicians encountered in beginning their careers in academic medicine. The change in the funding of science, coupled with inflation, gave students little hope for full-time academic careers. At the same time, the funds available for practice from Medicare, Medicaid, and third party payments increased.

The changes in funding for psychiatry were also having an effect on the feasibility of this career. The decreased funding for clinics and academic psychiatry by government and the effects of inflation made careers in these areas difficult. At the same time, there was an increasingly negative attitude by the public toward psychiatry, increased competition for private patients from psychologists and social workers, and only limited, if any, payment for psychiatry from Medicare, Medicaid, and third party payments. The decreased funding for public health also had an effect on students' career choices.

The increased difficulties in financing a medical education forced many students into the programs of the various armed services and the public health service, for which they received their medical education in return for four years of service. The impending federal manpower bill that would further control the type and geographical location of practice, although not law at that time, also had a marked effect on the students' career choices.

Within specialties such as surgery and diagnostic radiology, there were obviously too many practitioners, and this affected career choice. For example, the number of Harvard medical students choosing surgery as seniors was 24 percent in 1969 and 28 percent in 1970, but declined to 16 percent in 1973 and 12 percent in 1974. R.B. Freeman[7] has documented how quickly students respond to changes in the job market.

It was apparent to many students that many subspecialists could not devote themselves solely to their specialty and out of economic necessity devoted most of their time to primary care and only a small portion to their subspecialty. This was similar to the pattern of practice in the Specialty Era when most physicians in internal medicine practiced general internal medicine with attention to a subspecialty. As they grew older and their reputations grew, they eventually became subspecialists. During the Scientific Era this was reversed.

Equally apparent were the opportunities that were becoming available in primary care. The federal government encouraged physicians in this area, society demanded it, and third party payments now made such careers economically viable. The Robert Wood Johnson Foundation acted as a catalyst in the area of primary care.

Students' values were still a factor in their choice of family medicine. Within the bioscientific group, students frequently made the change to part-time academic medicine with a general internal medicine or general pediatric practice, which was more compatible with their values. Within both categories, over 90 percent wished to practice in groups, principally to reduce their hours of work and to allow them more time for other activities.

Although many factors were important in career choice during the Doldrums Era, undoubtedly the economic feasibility of careers was paramount. The deceased funding for academic medicine contributed to many shifts, and the increasing economic feasibility of careers in primary care made this career especially attractive.

The decline in the percentage of bioscientific students choosing full-time academic medicine continued during the Doldrums Era (see Figure 2-4). For the class of 1974, there was a 50 percent decrease between matriculation and graduation. Students planned careers in part-time academic medicine, although they still preferred full-time academic medicine. The major reason for the change was that students realized that funding was not available for such careers; also, they planned a more general type of specialty practice, this being more economically feasible.

Within the biosocial group, each year an increasing percentage of the students chose primary care, reaching 68 percent at graduation for the class of 1974. Psychiatry was chosen by 23 percent of the group, but public health as a career choice declined precipitously from its high of 38 percent in 1969 to 9 percent in 1974. This decline was related to the students finding that most public health positions were not action-oriented—"they research things to death" was the most frequent comment. The decline in funding was an added factor. In the class of 1974, between matriculation and graduation, family medicine increased from 58 percent to 68 percent and psychiatry from 15 percent to 22 percent while public health decreased from 26 percent to 10 percent.

The increase in the percentage choosing family medicine was related to the fact that it became a more viable career due to funding and current ideology. Increasingly, however, students chose general internal medicine or general pediatrics as their vehicle rather than general family medicine. The total percentage in psychiatry was far less than during the Scientific Era because far fewer students planning this career were admitted, or, if admitted, changed to family medicine. The student-practitioners, who in the past had switched to psychiatry because they saw family medicine as impractical during the Scientific Era, now saw it as possible and returned to their original plans. The decline in public health careers occurred because many students realized that the field was too research-oriented and too little action-oriented to suit their tastes. Then, too, students were less interested in social action. Decreased funding for these careers was also a factor.

THE PRIMARY CARE AND INCREASING GOVERNMENTAL CONTROL ERA

During 1975, at the beginning of the Primary Care and Increasing Governmental Control Era, the applicant pool remained large. There was a slight decrease in the number of minority group applicants, and the increase in women applicants continued. The grade point average (GPA) of all students continued to increase. The current pool contains so many academically able students that medical schools have a wide latitude in the admission of students with different career plans, different preparations, different socioeconomic backgrounds, minority status, and sex.

The type of student admitted continues to be predominantly bioscientific. The number of women and minority group students remains constant, and increasing numbers of these students are bioscientific. Within the biosocial group, the majority of students combine student-practitioner and student-psychiatrist characteristics. Few are admitted with the characteristics of one or the other. The GPAs and MCAT scores of students continue to increase.

The need for prestige and status remains high. Eighty-three percent would have chosen high prestige occupations had they not been admitted to medical school. The need for high financial rewards continues, especially among males, who expect to earn about $10,000 more per year than women. There is some decrease in the social commitment to change, with only 59 percent planning to be politically

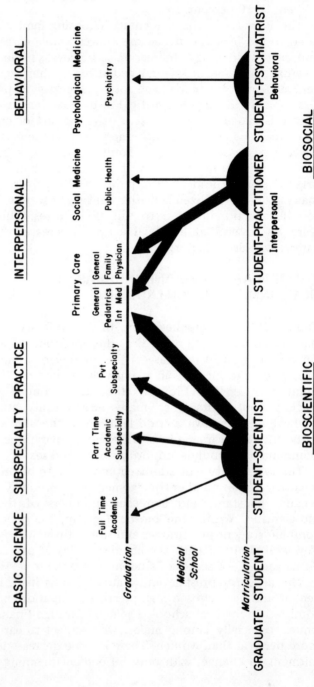

Figure 2-5. The Primary Care and Increasing Governmental Control Era—1975-
The thicker the line, the larger the number of students.

active on health issues. The social responsibility of the physician is first competence, with sizable numbers valuing the art of medicine and the delivery of care. Only 2 percent placed a top priority on research. There is less evidence of a preventive medicine or public health orientation in this era. Attitudes toward the elderly patient have improved, increasing to 48 percent with positive attitudes. However, the negative attitude toward patients with psychological symptoms continues. Although half of the students were bioscientific at matriculation, only 32 percent considered themselves in this category at graduation. There is a decrease in those students who consider themselves competitive, with the majority either equally competitive and cooperative or cooperative, which is consistent with valuing the delivery of medical care.

Ninety-five percent of the graduates plan to work in a group practice, the main reason being to have more time for their families and outside activities. Although the hours they expect to work are less for both men and women, the discrepancy continues between them, with an average of ten hours less for women. Women no longer feel that their lifestyle will inhibit their career plans. Their career choices differ little from those of men, except for a slightly higher percentage entering obstetrics and gynecology.

The decreased funding for academic medicine, research, and postdoctoral fellowships continues. It is apparent that well-trained physicians who are completing residencies and postdoctoral fellowships are having difficulties in securing academic positions as well as positions in specialties such as surgery. Many medical students who planned careers in academic medicine and surgery changed their career plans in medical school when they saw what was happening to recent graduates with these plans. The gap between faculty and students continues, with only 10 percent feeling that any role model in the medical school plays a part in their career choice.

Due to the loss of federal funding, careers in academic medicine have become difficult to pursue, and the increased third party payments have made more and more faculty dependent on their practices to sustain themselves. Certain specialties such as general surgery and diagnostic radiology are oversubscribed, making positions in these areas difficult to obtain. It is also evident that in many geographic areas there are too many practitioners. Ophthalmology, which is a shortage specialty, attracted eighteen students in the class of 1977 at Harvard Medical School, whereas in the past, only one or two students each year had chosen this specialty. Due to the decrease in the birth rate, some students are concerned with the economic viability of careers in pediatrics and obstetrics. The increasing number of empty beds in children's and lying-in hospitals contributes to their concern.

Nationally, there has been significant movement toward primary care. In a national sample of students at graduation in 1975, 45.5 percent elected primary care as compared to 54.8 percent at matriculation. As a percentage of the total class at graduation, 16.6 percent chose family medicine, 18.5 percent general internal medicine, and 10.4 percent general pediatrics. At matriculation, the percentages were 24.9 percent, 19.1 percent and 10.8 percent respectively (see Table 2-2).

Table 2-3 shows the percentages of the primary care specialties expressed as part of the total number in primary care. General internal medicine was the leading choice of graduates, but family practice was the leading choice of matriculating students in 1975. This upward trend has continued, since 60 percent of students in 1977 were matched for their first postgraduate year (internship) in primary care specialities.[8] Figure 2-5 shows the changes.

TRANSITIONAL PERIODS FROM ERA TO ERA

Much can be learned from the data on students during the transitional periods from one era to another. The contrast between the transition

Table 2-2. Career Choices of Medical Students in a National Representative of Medical Schools in 1975 at Graduation and Matriculation

	Graduation June 1975 Class of 1975		Matriculation September 1975 Class of 1979	
	N	%	N	%
Specialty				
General (family) practice	79 =	16.6	301 =	24.9
General internal medicine	87 =	18.5	231 =	19.1
General pediatrics	49 =	10.4	130 =	10.8
Total in primary care	214 =	45.5	662 =	54.8
Other specialties	257 =	54.5	547 =	45.2
Grand Totals:	471* =	100	1209+ =	100

*Eight respondents out of 479 failed to indicate a specialty choice.
+Thirty-three respondents out of 1,242 failed to indicate a specialty choice.

Table 2-3. The Percentage in the Specialties of Primary Care of Medical Students in a National Representative Sample of Medical Schools in 1975 at Graduation and Matriculation

	Graduation June 1975 Class of 1975		Matriculation September 1975 Class of 1979	
	N	%	*N*	%
Primary care subdivisions:				
General (family) practice	78 =	36.4	301 =	45.4
General internal medicine	87 =	40.6	231 =	34.8
General pediatrics	49 =	22.8	130 =	19.6
Totals:	214 =	100	662 =	100
Percent of class in primary care		50.0		58.1

from the Specialty to the Scientific Era in 1959-1961 and the current transition from the Doldrums into the Primary Care and Increasing Governmental Control Era is significant despite the similarities.

In the transition from the Specialty to the Scientific Era, faculty, students, government, foundations, and society embraced the change. Students who entered medical school in the Specialty Era and who were bioscientific easily adjusted and quickly changed from planning part-time to planning full-time academic careers, which they preferred. Student-practitioners, the largest subgroup of biosocial students, reacted to the change in three different ways: one group changed their characteristics in medical school to those of the bioscientific students, chose such careers at graduation, and were happy and effective; another group compromised by choosing psychiatry, which was adequately funded and thus gave them the opportunity to continue to work directly with people; a small group, unable to change or compromise, chose either general practice, a general specialty, or academic medicine, but were extremely bitter and unhappy with their choice.[9]

In the current transition into the Primary Care and Increasing Governmental Control Era, there are several differences. The great majority of faculty members are opposed to the change as they see in it the decline of funding for science. The students are divided as to the merits of the new era depending upon their career plans, and society and the government are pressing for the new era.

This time it is the bioscientific students who are having difficulty in career choices. The biosocial students are supported by society and by the government as they plan careers in primary care, particularly family medicine. Bioscientific students still prefer full-time academic subspecialty careers with research. They are handling the forced career change by the same three mechanisms just described: either they are embracing the new primary care specialties, changing their characteristics and looking forward to a fruitful career, or they are compromising by practicing a primary care specialty—most often in general internal medicine with special attention to a subspecialty, with the hope that as they grow older, they can become subspecialists. The third group of students are entering a specialty that they did not originally plan or prefer, and are now unhappy and angry.

❋   *Chapter 3*

Changes in Career Choices: A Chronological Basis

AN OVERVIEW

The changes in the career choices of medical students from matriculation to graduation during various eras of medicine have been described. These data will now be considered in a different context.

Examining the data of freshmen and seniors in the same chronological year makes it possible to test the following hypothesis: when societal factors change, the career choices of matriculating and graduating students change simultaneously in the same chronological year. If the data support this hypothesis, the predominant role of societal factors in career choices will be confirmed.

Figure 3-1 shows the changes in the career choices of matriculating and graduating students arranged chronologically. Students were classified as biosocial, bioscientific, or bioengineering. Data were collected on students at the end of their sophomore years in 1960, 1961, 1970, and 1971.

A limited sample of students' career choices during the Specialty Era were obtained by examining admissions and graduation records of the classes from 1947 through 1959. Because these data were obtained by a retrospective technique, they are not shown on the graph, but will be discussed.

First, the changes in career orientation between 1958 and 1970 will be discussed, later the changes subsequent to this will be detailed. It is striking that from 1958 to 1970, the changes in career orientations, whether primarily bioscientific or biosocial, occurred simul-

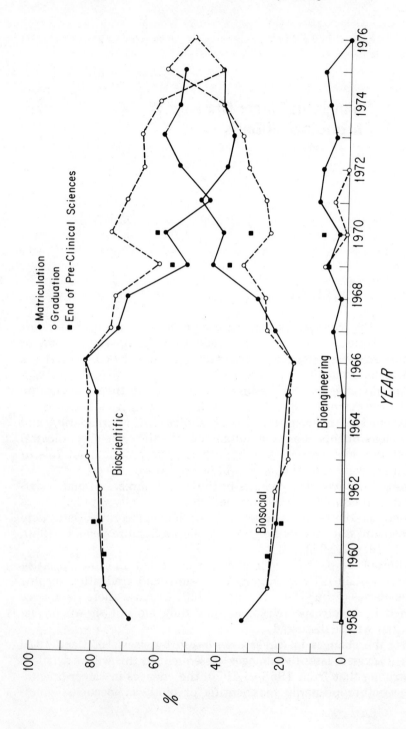

Figure 3-1. Harvard Medical Students' Career Plans

taneously in freshmen, sophomores, and seniors. Additionally, the changes are limited to the two transitions from the Specialty to the Scientific Era and from the Scientific to the Student Activism Era. Changes do not occur during the stable Specialty and Scientific Eras. For example, in 1959, with the onset of the Scientific Era, large numbers of freshmen and seniors changed to bioscientifically oriented careers characteristic of this era, whereas the seniors and freshmen of the previous year had shown the career choices of the Specialty Era. Again, in 1967, when the transition period toward a Student Activism Era began, with a decrease in the number choosing bioscientific careers and an increase in those choosing biosocial careers, the change occurred simultaneously in both freshmen and seniors. When this trend reached its peak in 1969, the changes were concomitant in freshmen, sophomores, and seniors. In 1970, when a trend away from the career orientations characteristic of the Student Activism Era began, with an increase in the percentage of students electing bioscientific careers and a decrease in those selecting biosocial careers, these changes took place in all three classes in that year.

In contrast to this, between 1959 and 1967, when medicine was in the stable Scientific Era, there was little change in any year in either the entering or graduating classes. A retrospective study of the classes from 1947 to 1959, during the stable Specialty Era, showed little change in career orientations in any year in either the entering or graduating classes.

The changes occurring in career orientations during transition periods, but not during stable eras, were paralleled by the changes in the same periods in other data collected on this project. These data show extensive changes in premedical preparation, attitudes, values, and measured interests during transition periods, but only minor changes during the stable eras. For example, an analysis of the premedical college preparation of students during the Specialty Era showed that the majority majored in either general science (premedical) or the humanities. With the change to the Scientific Era, the premedical majors rapidly declined to zero and the humanities majors from 40 percent to less than 20 percent. Most students majored in biology or chemistry. Many students secured advanced standing in science in college and studied graduate courses as undergraduates. Once this new pattern of premedical preparation was established, except for a gradual increase in the amount of science studied and the addition of mathematics and physics majors later in the era, there was little change.

With the onset of the next transition, from the Scientific Era to the Student Activism Era in 1967, the premedical preparation of students changed. This time, the change was toward studying the social sciences more appropriate to community interests. In the classes entering from 1958 through 1967, approximately 20 percent of the students in each class had taken a social science course in college. In 1968, this changed abruptly. Seventy-four percent of the class that entered had taken a social science course. This increased in subsequent classes until it reached 92 percent for the class that entered in 1970, and it has since continued at this level.

The abrupt changes in premedical preparation in the first transition era in 1958 and in the one that began in 1967 are particularly interesting if the transcripts of premedical students in all four college classes at that time are examined. It was in 1959 that premedical students who would become applicants to the Harvard Medical School began to study more science and to change their majors from nonscience to science and from premedical majors to biology or chemistry. In 1959, this change occurred in premedical students who were seniors, juniors, sophomores, or freshmen.

The same, simultaneous change in all four college classes who would apply to Harvard Medical School occurred again in 1968, but this time it was away from the natural sciences toward the study of the social and behavioral sciences. Examination of the college transcripts of students who would apply to the Harvard Medical School showed that simultaneously seniors, juniors, sophomores, and freshmen substituted social or behavioral science for natural science courses in 1968. The pool of applicants to the Harvard Medical School represents a diverse distribution of colleges nationally. Simultaneously, in 1959 and 1968, premedical students in all four classes in such different colleges as Bowdoin, Harvard, Yale, Swarthmore, Texas, Florida, Stanford, Chicago, Nebraska, and Washington all moved in the same direction—toward science in the first instance, away from it in the second.

These data are especially important if they are related to changes in the career choices of medical students. In the 1959–1960 academic year, when the premedical students in all four college classes nationwide were increasing their science preparation, Harvard medical students who were freshmen, sophomores, and seniors changed their career choices to those that were more bioscientifically oriented. Large numbers within the bioscientific group changed from private specialty practice to academic medicine. Sizable numbers of students within the medical school indicated on questionnaires that they wished they had studied more science in college. This was a new phenomenon.

In 1968, when premedical students in all four college classes nationwide were substituting social and behavioral science courses for courses in the natural sciences, Harvard medical freshmen, sophomores, and seniors were changing their career choices toward those more socially oriented. Within the biosocial group, large numbers moved from psychiatry to public health and family medicine. For the first time, sizable numbers of these students indicated on questionnaires that if they could return to college they would change their premedical preparation to include more of the social and behavioral sciences.

Examination of the changes since 1970 shows a slight difference in the changes in the freshmen and the seniors (see Figure 3-1). However, the trend is the same, with a decline in bioscientific careers and an increase in biosocial careers, so that by 1975-1976, each class is almost equally divided between the two. Through the period of the seventies, the changes in the career choices of freshmen and seniors in the same year were parallel.

ANALYSES OF FINDINGS

These data are interpreted as indicating that the career orientations and preparation of students are more related to factors outside the medical school than within it. Otherwise, there is no plausible explanation why the entering freshman, sophomore, and senior medical students as well as college students in all four classes who would eventually become Harvard medical applicants—all showed the same changes simultaneously in 1959 and 1968. It was not the effect of a change in admissions policy, because an analysis of the pool of applicants to each class slows that those selected did not differ significantly from the unsuccessful applicants on these variables.

The many factors that facilitated the transition from the Specialty to the Scientific Era were clearly a part of national policy. However, the factors that ignited student activism are not clear, since the change was not in line with national policy, nor was it encouraged by colleges, universities, or medical schools. Thus, although the changes in premedical preparation and in career choices were looked upon by the majority of students as individual choices, the fact that they were made by so many, across such a wide spectrum, argues against this rationale. It is much more likely that these decisions were made in response to other factors affecting the mass of students.

During the Doldrums Era, students were subjected to new societal factors: the cuts in research funds and fellowships, making a career in academic medicine difficult; the efforts by society and Congress to force more students into primary care with the impending Manpower Act; and the strong drive by medical school faculty to increase the number of students electing bioscientific careers. Evidence of this faculty effort was seen in (1) the attempt to change the pass-fail system adopted in the Student Activism Era back to a letter grading system because "competition was the lifeblood of science,"[1] (2) the adoption of the first M.D.-Ph.D. program, and (3) the increased number of basic scientists volunteering to serve on admission committees.

The mixture of societal factors, some from outside the medical school and others from within, affected students' career choices. Outside the medical school, these factors included the impending federal legislation mandating a certain percentage of students to enter primary care as well as the demands by society for primary care physicians; the decreased funding for science, making careers in academic medicine difficult; and oversubscription in certain specialties such as surgery and subspecialty medicine. At the same time, the decreased funds for science resulted in an increase in bioscientific applicants. This was due to the fact that many students who had entered college planning to go to graduate school switched to mediicine. Many graduate students and Ph.Ds in science, acting under the same economic pressures, applied to medical schools in increasing numbers.

Within the medical schools, the pressure from the basic science faculty for the admittance of more student-scientists resulted early in the era in many freshmen choosing bioscientific careers. But late in the era, pressures from minority group students and women for admission resulted in many more choosing primary care. As the result of these pressures, early in the era almost all bioscientific students admitted were majority males; almost all biosocial students were minority group students or women. Late in the era, the bioscientific students continued to be predominantly majority males, but slowly the percentage of minority group and women bioscientific students increased. The increase in bioscientific minority students was due to the fact than an increased number of them had been accepted into colleges or universities with outstanding science departments. The increase in bioscientific women occurred because many of those who had entered college planning to go to graduate school later switched to medicine because science no longer seemed economically viable.

The pressures of the basic science faculty to secure students who would choose bioscientific careers resulted in the increased selection of those who were thought to have the best chance of electing such careers. There was an increase in the admission of students who had entered college planning to go to graduate school in the sciences but who had switched to medicine. These data show the increased selection of such students; hence it is not surprising that the percentage of entering students choosing bioscientific careers was approximately 50 percent. However, these data also show that at admission, a far higher percentage indicated bioscientific career choices than did at matriculation a year later. The applicants obviously knew what the medical school admissions committees wanted to hear.

At the end of the Doldrums Era in 1974, with the impending Primary Care and Increasing Governmental Control Era, there was again, just as in other transitional periods, a dramatic change in the career orientations of students. There was an abrupt decline in the seniors choosing bioscientific careers, down from 58 percent in 1974 to 42 percent in 1975. Concomitantly, there was an increase in those choosing biosocial careers, from 40 percent in 1974 to 48 percent in 1975. For the first time in our studies of medical students from 1947 to 1976, the percentage of students choosing biosocial careers equaled or exceeded those choosing bioscientific careers.

This project terminated; hence we have no data on the matriculating students in 1976. Of the matriculating students in 1975, 52 percent chose bioscientific careers, with 40 percent biosocial and 8 percent bioengineering. It is remarkable that the percentage of those planning biosocial careers was this high because of the efforts of the faculty to admit bioscientific students and the increasing numbers of students admitted who had entered college planning to go to graduate school in the sciences but later changed to medicine. Even so, 42 percent of first year students opting for biosocial careers was an increase from the 17 percent in 1966, the height of the Scientific Era. The effect of admissions policy can also be seen in the fact that the percentage of students choosing bioscientific careers at admissions was considerably higher than when these data were collected on the same students at matriculation.

BIOSCIENTIFIC CAREERS

A further dimension in understanding the changes in the career choices of students can be seen by examining the data on the specific career choices within the bioscientific group chronologically from 1958 to 1976.

Figures 3–2 and 3–3 show the career plans of students within the bioscientific group at matriculation and at graduation, calculated separately for each class and categorized on the following basis: (1) part-time faculty, clinical specialty; (2) full-time medical faculty,

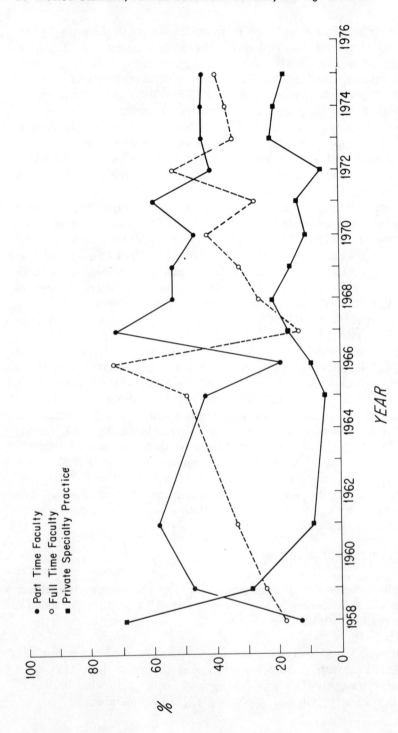

Figure 3-2.   Harvard Medical Students Planning Bioscientific Careers at Matriculation

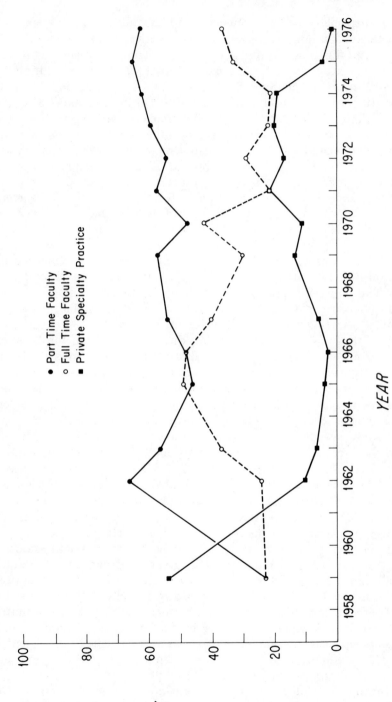

Figure 3-3.   Harvard Medical Students Planning Bioscientific Careers at Graduation

clinical specialty or basic sciences; and (3) full-time private specialty practice, excluding psychiatry, family practice, and public health.

Within the bioscientific group, the matriculating and graduating students show dramatic changes in their career plans during the transition from the Specialty to the Scientific Era and from the Scientific to the Student Activism Era. During the stable Specialty and Scientific Eras, there were less dramatic changes in the career choices of students. During the Doldrums Era, both freshmen and seniors indicated part-time academic medicine as their first choice.

During the stable Specialty Era, 1947–1958, 70 percent of the students chose private specialty practice, with part-time and full-time academic medicine accounting for the remaining 30 percent. Many students in this group preferred full-time academic careers but did not see such careers as financially viable. In truth, they were not.

With the onset of the transition from the Specialty to the Scientific Era in the fall of 1959, there was a rapid increase among both matriculating and graduating students in the percentage of each class choosing academic careers with a concomitant fall in the percentage selecting private specialty practice.

During the stable Scientific Era, the changes within the bioscientific group were consistent with what would be expected as the era gradually came into full bloom. During the early 1960s, the majority of students planned part-time academic careers, but by 1965, when the era was at its zenith, most planned full-time academic careers. This change occurred because it was possible to study science on a more advanced level in secondary school, college, and medical school, and the increasing funds for research made full-time academic medicine a viable career option. Only 5 percent of the class that entered in 1959 were undecided between an M.D. and a Ph.D.; in 1965, 48 percent of the matriculants were struggling with this dilemma.

In 1967, when the transitional era from the Scientific to the Student Activism Era began, the number of students electing full-time academic medicine decreased in both freshmen and seniors at the same time. This reduction was greater in matriculants than in graduates. From 1968 to 1971, the percentage of each class choosing full-time academic medicine increased marginally, but was far below the percentage at the height of the Scientific Era. By 1971, at matriculation and at graduation, the percentage choosing full-time academic careers was less than one-half of those at the height of the Scientific Era. At graduation, the decrease was from 48 percent to 22 percent; at matriculation, from 74 percent to 27 percent.

During the Doldrums Era, the percentage within the bioscientific group at matriculation and at graduation remained constant. At the close of the Doldrums in 1974 and the beginning of the new era in 1975, there was little change within the bioscientific choice of careers except for an increase within the group of those choosing full-time academic medicine at graduation. The reason for this was the marked decrease in the percentage of students choosing bioscientific careers. The increased percentage of students is based on the smaller number of students in this category. Actually, it represents a decrease in absolute numbers from twenty to nineteen over the three year period.

The data on the bioscientific students parallel the data reported on the career orientations of the classes as a whole. Within the bioscientific group, changes occurred simultaneously in freshmen and seniors, indicating the importance of influences outside of the medical school. Again, noticeable changes occurred in the two transition periods, with less dramatic changes during the stable Specialty, Scientific, and Doldrums Eras.

At the beginning of the transition era in 1967, the fall in the percentage of students choosing full-time academic careers paralleled the decrease in bioscientific and the increase in biosocial career orientations already reported. Again, the changes within the bioscientific group in 1967 away from full-time academic careers, as well as changes in the class as a whole, occurred in both freshmen and seniors and at the same time.

Since 1971, the percentage of students choosing full-time academic careers has remained constant, but is considerably less than one-half of the percentage who chose such careers at the height of the Scientific Era. Although students still prefer this career, they choose part-time academic medicine. The numbers choosing full-time academic careers at matriculation were considerably greater than those at graduation. This was due to the admission of more students who preferred graduate school to medical school but who switched to the latter because it was more viable. Hence, the decrease between matriculation and graduation in the number of seniors planning full-time academic medicine was due to the more realistic appraisal by the seniors of the funding for full-time academic careers, although they still preferred such careers.

BIOSOCIAL CAREERS

The effect of societal factors on the career choices of students is even more apparent in biosocial careers. Figures 3-4 and 3-5 show the career plans of students within the biosocial group at matriculation and at graduation chronologically from 1958 to 1976 categorized

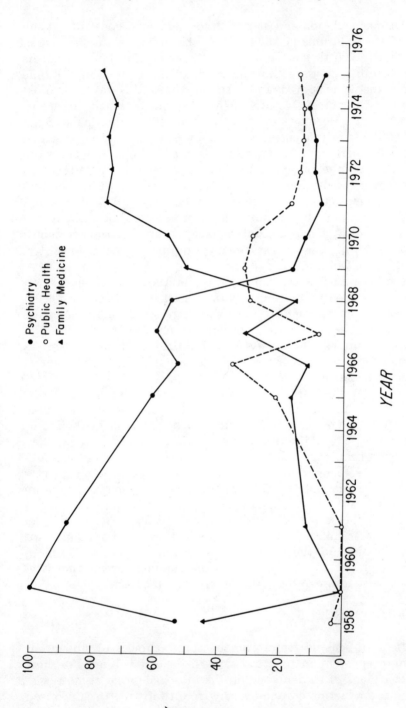

Figure 3–4.   Harvard Medical Students Planning Biosocial Careers at Matriculation

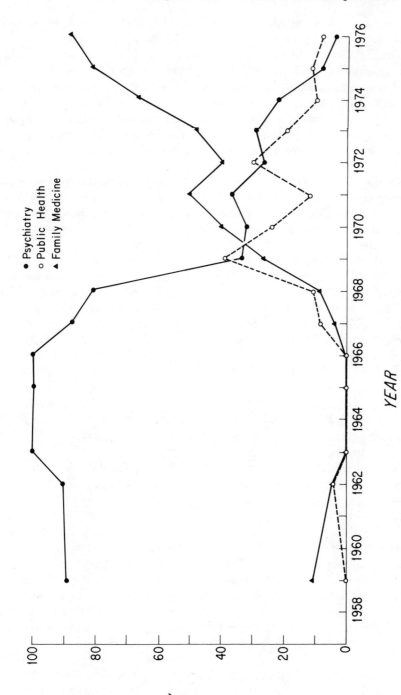

Figure 3-5. Harvard Medical Students at Graduation Planning Biosocial Careers

on the following bases: (1) psychiatry, (2) public health associated with the delivery of medical care, and (3) family medicine.

During the stable Specialty and Scientific Eras, the matriculating and graduating students within the biosocial group showed changes that were gradual and consistent with the new opportunities offered by the eras. During the transition from the Specialty to the Scientific Era and from the Scientific to the Student Activism Era, the changes were sudden and significant. The Student Activism Era, only two years long, never stabilized; changes during the longer Doldrums Era were gradual.

During the Specialty Era, the retrospective data showed that approximately 40-45 percent of matriculants chose general practice, and by graduation, 15-20 percent still planned to follow this career. The remainder chose careers in general pediatrics or general internal medicine.

During the transition from the Specialty to the Scientific Era, the rapidity of change within the biosocial group can be seen in the following data. The last class in the Specialty Era matriculated in 1959, at which time 44 percent of this group planned careers in general practice; the next class entered at the start of the Scientific Era contained no students planning this career. Eleven percent of the last class to graduate in the Specialty Era (1959) planned to become general practitioners; in 1962, it was 4 percent, and by 1963, zero.

In contrast to the marked, sudden changes in the transition period, the changes were minimal and uniform as the Scientific Era stabilized between 1959 and 1967. In each matriculating class, only a small number planned careers in general practice; by graduation, all had decided to become psychiatrists.

The transition from the Scientific to the Student Activism Era became evident in the biosocial group with changes in the career plans of freshmen in 1966 and seniors in 1967. There was a dramatic increase in the numbers planning careers in family medicine and public health, and a dramatic fall in those choosing psychiatry. These changes were marked from 1966 through 1968, but accelerated dramatically from 1968 to 1969.

The brief 1969-1970 Student Activism Era never stabilized. In 1969, public health, which was perceived as enabling a physician to be active against the social factors impeding health and causing disease, was chosen by the highest percentage of biosocial seniors. By 1971, at the beginning of the Doldrums Era, the choice of public health had fallen noticeably, and family medicine had risen to 76 percent of matriculants and 49 percent of graduates. During the remainder of the era, the career choices of matriculating students remained constant; among seniors, there was a gradual increase in family medicine to 81 percent, with the decline in psychiatry and public health continuing.

In 1975, at the beginning of the Primary Care and Increasing Governmental Control Era, 88 percent of the seniors in the biosocial group elected family medicine, with only 4 percent electing psychiatry, which had been 100 percent during most of the Scientific Era. Public health had fallen to 8 percent.

Comment

Viewing these data on career choices classified as bioscientific or biosocial and within each of these classifications in a longitudinal, chronological manner in both matriculating and graduating students highlights the importance of societal factors. The changes in freshmen, in seniors, and, on the two occasions where there are data, in sophomores, occurred in all three medical school classes simultaneously. Parallel with this, in the same year of the transition to the Scientific Era, college students in each class—freshmen, sophomores, juniors, and seniors—throughout the nation began to study more science. Again, in 1968-1969, in the transition to the Student Activism Era, college students in each class nationwide began to study more social science. These parallel changes on two separate occasions in matriculating, second year, and graduating medical students as well as in students in all four years of college nationwide are evidence of the importance of societal factors.

The effect of societal factors can be seen clearly if we look at three different career choices over the years; full-time academic medicine, psychiatry, and family medicine. About 18-20 percent of matriculating and graduating students during the Specialty Era planned full-time careers in academic medicine, although a much higher percentage preferred it. At the height of the Scientific Era, over 50 percent of seniors and 70 percent of freshmen in the bioscientific group opted for this career. With the change in ideology and eventually the decreased funding, this percentage fell to a low of 27 percent in freshmen and 22 percent in seniors. The gradual increase since then to 39 percent of freshmen and 36 percent of seniors actually represents no change in absolute numbers because of the small numbers choosing bioscientific careers.

During the Specialty Era, there was a gradual increase in those choosing psychiatry as a career because of National Institute of Mental Health funding, and society's approval. Psychiatry reached its peak during the Scientific Era, with all Harvard Medical School seniors in the biosocial group choosing this career. Many originally chose general practice, but as the result of their medical school experience saw psychiatry as the only remaining opportunity to work on a close interpersonal basis with patients. Freshmen in 1966 and seniors in 1967 began to choose psychiatry less often; by 1969, combining freshmen, sophmores, and senior career choices, only 23 percent elected psychiatry. By 1976, the percentage of seniors had fallen to 4 percent.

General practice was the choice of 40–45 percent of matriculating students and 15–20 percent of graduating students during the Specialty Era. However, only 10–15 percent of entering students chose this career during the Scientific Era; by graduation, none elected general practice. Instead, they chose psychiatry. Once the Student Activism Era was underway, the changes were dramatic. The percentage of biosocial students choosing family medicine rose from zero at graduation in 1966 to 88 percent at graduation in 1976. Only 18 percent chose biosocial careers at graduation in 1966, of which 100 percent were in psychiatry; in 1976, at graduation, 50 percent chose biosocial careers, 88 percent being in family medicine, 4 percent in psychiatry.

Chapter 4

Primary Care

PRIMARY CARE IN THE VARIOUS ERAS

One of the objectives of this study was to analyze characteristics of students and physicians who plan to make their
careers in primary care. The general use of the term primary care is
new. The term, used to describe the vehicle of primary care as well
as the tasks assigned to practitioners of primary care, has changed
with each era. When this study began nineteen years ago during the
Specialty Era, the vehicle was general practice. During the Scientific
Era, when subspecialty practice was the choice of most students at
graduation, there were too few general practitioners to warrant study.
However, during that era, sufficient numbers of students planning to
become general practitioners matriculated so that studies could be
made of the changes in their career plans during medical school. In
the Student Activism Era and during the early years of the Doldrums
Era, family medicine became the vehicle for this type of practice.
Currently, primary care as defined by the Manpower Act of 1976
encompasses family medicine, general internal medicine, and general
pediatrics. For the purposes of this research, the characteristics and
changes during medical school of those electing careers in primary
care encompass the group of students planning to practice using the
vehicle appropriate to each era.

The Specialty Era

The students who became general practitioners during the Specialty Era of the fifties has characteristics of the student-practi-

tioner.[1] Their chief interest was to work directly with people, using science pragmatically to solve medical problems. Compared with other medical students, they had lower grades, lower Medical College Admission Test scores, and less science preparation. On the Strong Vocational Interest Blank, they had measured interests in working directly with people but did not show measured interests in the sciences or in human behavior. They were concerned with individual patients, were not interested in social factors, and did not have a public health orientation. These characteristics were also found in the Association of American Medical Colleges study of students who graduated in 1960 in a national stratified sample of medical schools,[2] by Sanazaro in a national study of house officers,[3] and by Lyden, Geiger, and Peterson in their study of physicians.[4]

The Scientific Era

During the Scientific Era of the sixties, the data are inconclusive because the number choosing the primary care specialty of general practice was too small. However, those with the characteristics of student-practitioners at matriculation planned careers in general practice early in the era. By graduation, however, all of these at Harvard Medical School had changed to psychiatry. They perceived medicine as too technological and saw the psychiatrist as the only physician who still had close personal contact with patients.[5] Some of the data show that this shift into psychiatry was somewhat less apparent at medical schools lacking strong psychiatry departments and where the number of psychiatrists per capita within that state was small.[6] Again, the importance of societal factors in career choice was evident.

The Student Activism Era

During the brief era of student activism, there was a revival of interest in primary care, principally in family medicine. The American Board of Family Practice was established in 1969. Students at this time were intensely interested in social activism and in using medicine to change society. They had a strong public health orientation and placed their highest value on the delivery of medical care to deprived areas, without cost to patients.

Almost all of the biosocial students shifted from psychiatry to family medicine or public health. They saw this latter specialty as providing the opportunity to be socially active in medicine. A few of the bioscientific students shifted their career plans to family medicine or public health, especially at the end of their second year in medical school.

The data show that many of these students saw a medical education as a means to change society. They would discard the scientific analyses of problems before taking action and would use trial and error to solve the problems of medical care delivery. Students entering in 1969 had markedly increased their study of the social sciences during their last year in college; those matriculating in 1970 had a similar increase during their last two years of college.

The Doldrums Era

The period of student activism was over by 1971. The career choices of students early in the Doldrums Era differed from those late in the era, when the harbingers of the new Primary Care and Increasing Governmental Control Era appeared.

Early in the era, before the societal and ideological forces of the next era were apparent, it was possible to examine the characteristics of students who were committed to primary care as family physicians. This was not possible late in the era because of the mass stampede into primary care by both biosocial and bioscientific students. Early in the era students, for reasons of interest, basic personality needs, and personal characteristics, entered primary care. Late in the era and also in the next era, these same students were joined by many bioscientific students who would have preferred bioscientific careers, particularly in subspecialty medicine, but who no longer thought such careers viable due to the decreased funding of academic medicine and the increasing number of subspecialists.

To illustrate the characteristics of students choosing careers related to primary care during the Doldrums, analyses of the data were made of the Harvard Medical School classes of 1971, 1972, and 1973, and of the University of Michigan Medical School class of 1973. The basic characteristics of these students at admissions and matriculation, as well as their grades on the National Board of Medical Examinations, Parts I and II, were compared with their choice of careers at graduation.

The career choices at graduation were classified as bioscientific or biosocial as established by previous criteria. The analyses would have been more accurate had the careers at graduation been classified as family medicine or other. Regardless, 82 percent of the biosocial careers choices were family medicine, 11 percent public health, and 8 percent psychiatry. A followup study of these students three years later showed 92 percent of them in family practice. Thus, almost all of the biosocial group are family practitioners who are delivering primary care.

Table 4-1 shows that when students were classified as bioscientific

Table 4-1. The Predicted Versus Actual Career Choices for Harvard and Michigan Medical Students, Harvard Medical School classes of 1971, 1972, 1973, and Michigan Medical School class of 1973

Predicted career orientation at matriculation	*Actual Career Orientation at Graduation*		
	Bioscientific	*Biosocial*	
Bioscientific	122 (48.8%)	26 (10.4%)	148 (59.2%)
Biosocial	33 (13.2%)	69 (27.6%)	102 (40.8%)
Totals	155 (62.0%)	95 (38.0%)	250

Chi square = 62.171   Sig. under 0.001 with one degree of freedom

Therefore, the number of correct predictions is: (122 + 69) = 191 (76.4%). If we had predicted at random, the chances would be 50/50 that we would predict correctly. Consequently, we have improved our predictive accuracy from 50% to 76.4%:

This initial corrected regression uses only the limited number of variables.

1. Matriculation Questionnaire Career Orientation (Bioscientific = 0, Biosocial = 1)
2. Quantitative MCAT
3. Preference for working in family practice community medicine as opposed to private specialty practice, research, public health, etc. (1 = highest, 6 = lowest)
4. Whether the respondent considered law as a serious possible alternative to medicine
5. Whether the respondent considered psychology as a serious possible alternative to medicine
6. How highly the respondent considered monetary values in his choice of medicine as a career

The overall equation for prediction is:

Predict = 1.756 = .3245*(1) - .0016*(2) - .0695*(3) - .1849*(4) - .1871*(5) + .0921*(6)

or biosocial on the basis of admission and matriculation data, four years later at graduation, bioscientific students chose bioscientific careers and biosocial students chose biosocial careers at a highly significant level. This was determined by regression analysis. The most predictive variables for a bioscientific career at matriculation were that students considered themselves primarily scientifically oriented, had high quantitative scores on the Medical College Admission Test, had actually planned a bioscientific career, had not considered law or psychology as alternative careers, and placed a high value on monetary rewards. In contrast to this, biosocial students considered themselves primarily "people-oriented," had lower quantitative MCAT scores, planned family practice or public health careers, had considered law or psychology as alternate careers, and placed a low value on monetary rewards. There were also other significant indicators. This shows that it was possible during 1971, 1972, and 1973 to predict at a highly significant level the career choices of students at graduation from admission and matriculation data.

Another method of analyzing these same data was to classify students in bioscientific or biosocial careers at graduation and to relate these choices to their admission and matriculation data. It will be recalled that over 92 percent of the students classified as biosocial were, in fact, in family medicine. Striking and significant differences emerged between the two groups on the admission and matriculation data (see Table 4-2).

Students choosing bioscientific careers were predominantly male, came from families with high incomes, had high MCAT quantitative and science scores, had majored in science, had taken more science courses from which they derived their greatest satisfaction, had made high grades in science, had measured interests in science, admired Einstein, had spent more than one summer doing research, rated scientific work and research high in their career choice, and expected to spend time in research. They predicted the clinical years to be the most difficult. In values, they gave high priority to status, income, and scientific research. They were conservative in that they did not rate changing society as important, would retain fee for service, and did not consider participation in community affairs important. They scored higher than biosocial students in every subject on the National Board of Medical Examinations, Parts I and II, except psychiatry.

Students choosing biosocial careers were more apt to be female, to come from families with moderate incomes, to have lower science and quantitative MCAT scores, to be nonscience majors with many courses in psychology and government, to derive their greatest pleasure from behavioral and social science courses, to have measured interests in interpersonal or human behavior, to rate interpersonal relationships high, to not be research-oriented, and to emphasize patient care. They had considered law or psychology as alternate careers and felt that the first year would be the most difficult. They were social activists and wanted to change society, participate in community affairs, and abolish fee for service. Only in psychiatry did they score higher on the national boards than the bioscientific students. The nonprimary care physician showed the characteristics of the student-scientist; the primary care physician showed character-

Table 4-2. Summary of a Sample of the Data. University of Michigan Medical School Class 1973; Harvard Medical School Classes—1971, 1972, 1973

Matriculation Data	Careers at Graduation	
	Bioscientific	Biosocial
I. Basic characteristics		
A. Personal data		
Sex	Male	Female
Parent's annual income	High	Low to moderate
B. Aptitudes		
MCAT quantitative scores	Very high	Moderate
MCAT science scores	High	Moderate
C. Preparation		
Undergraduate major	Science	Nonscience
Number of semesters of undergraduate chemistry	Many	Few
Number of semesters of undergraduate physics	More than minimal requirements	Minimal requirements
Number of semesters of undergraduate biophysics	Some	None
Number of semesters of undergraduate psychology	Few	Many
Number of semesters of undergraduate political science or government	Few	Many
Adequacy of college education for a career in medicine	Very adequate	Merely adequate to inadequate
D. Interests		
Rating of importance of social sciences	Low	High
Rating of importance of natural sciences	High	Low
Rating of importance of behavioral sciences	Low	Higher
Undergraduate grades in natural sciences	High	Moderate
Undergraduate grades in social sciences	Low	High
Measured interest in human behavior on SVIB	Low	High
Importance of intellectual tasks as compared with interpersonal relations and introspection in their medical practice	High	Low

Importance of interpersonal relations in their medical practice	Moderate	High
Admiration of Einstein as compared with Churchill and Freud	High	Moderate
Numbers of summers spent in a research-oriented job	More than one	One
Rate "Doing work that involved scientific method and research" as factors in career choice	High	Low
Rate "Importance of being able to work with people rather than things" as factor in selection of career of medicine	Low	High
Percentage of time expected to spend in teaching	High	Low
Percentage of time expected to spend in administration	Low	High
Percentage of time expected to spend in patient care	Low	High
Percentage of time wanted to spend in research	High	Low
Percentage of time wanted to spend in administration	Low	High
Considered any profession other than medicine as serious possible alternative?	No	Yes
In particular, considered business	Yes	No
In particular, considered teaching in college	No	Yes
In particular, considered law	No	Yes
In particular, considered psychology	No	Yes
Doubts about becoming a doctor after decision to go to medical school had been made	None	Some
Year predicted to be hardest at medical school	Clinical years	First year

II. Values

Importance of status, income, and scientific research as factors in choice of medicine as a career	High	Low
Personal feelings toward sick people who are down and out	Neutral	Positive
Rating of "being able to change society" as factor in career choice	Not important	Important

Table 4-2 continued

Rating of "participation in community affairs" as worthwhile postgraduate activity	Not important	Important
Should "fee for service" be retained for the majority of physicians	Yes	No
Should "fee for service" be retained for the respondent	Yes	No
III. Lifestyle		
Consideration of "group practice with salary" as mode of practice	Less favored	Favored
IV Achievement in medical school		
National Board (NBME) scores on: Anatomy, Physiology, Biochemistry, Pathology, Microbiology, Pharmacology, PART I Totals, Medicine, Surgery, Obstetrics, PART II Totals Psychiatry	High Moderate	Lower Higher

Table 4-2 continued

Matriculation Data	Careers at Graduation				
	Bioscientific Mean	N	Biosocial Mean	N	Sig
I. Basic characteristics					
A. Personal data					
Sex: 1=male, 2=female	1.000	36	1.111	36	0.041
Majority=minority status: 1=majority, 2=minority	1.028	72	1.135	37	0.031
Parent's annual income: 1=lowest interval, 2=highest interval	4.119	59	3.560	25	0.051
B. Aptitudes					
MCAT quantitative score	704.20	112	669.82	56	0.001
MCAT science score	654.55	112	625.89	56	0.001
C. Preparation					
Undergraduate major: 1=Biology, 2=Biochemistry, 3=Biophysics, 4=Chemistry, 5=Physical Science, 6=Social Science, 7=Psychology, 8=Humanities, 9=Premed or general science	3.485	103	4.980	50	0.002
College Major divided along science (=1) and nonscience (=2)					
Number of semesters of undergraduate chemistry	1.104	67	1.371	35	0.002
Number of semesters of undergraduate physics	7.452	42	5.905	21	0.021
Number of semesters of undergraduate biophysics	3.429	42	2.476	21	0.042
Number of semesters of undergraduate psychology	0.183	71	0.000	37	0.017
Number of semesters of undergraduate political science or government	1.296	71	2.757	37	0.009
	0.873	71	2.270	37	0.010
Rating of adequacy of college preparation for a medical career: 1=very adequate, 2=adequate, 3=inadequate	1.581	62	1.017	24	0.059

Table 4-2 continued

Matriculation Data	Careers at Graduation				
	Bioscientific Mean	N	Biosocial Mean	N	Sig
Rank personal pleasure derived from study of natural science: 1=most, 4=least	1.239	71	2.000	32	0.001
Rank personal pleasure derived from study of social science: 1=most, 4=least	3.361	61	2.667	24	0.002
Rank personal pleasure derived from study of behavioral science: 1=most, 4=least	2.652	69	1.937	32	0.001
Rank grades received as an undergraduate in natural science: 1=highest, 4=lowest	1.353	68	1.839	31	0.004
Rank grades received as an undergraduate in social science: 1=highest, 4=lowest	3.018	57	2.254	21	0.054
D. Interests					
Group X profile, interest in human behavior on Strong Vocational Interest Blank: 1 indicates a positive interest, 0 a negative or neutral interest	0.451	71	0.697	33	0.020
Group II summary, interest in science on Strong Vocation Interest Blank	44.239	71	36.970	33	0.001
Rank importance of intellectual tasks as compared with interpersonal relations and introspection: 1=highest value of the three, 3=lowest	1.674	98	2.106	47	0.001
Rank importance of interpersonal relations in same list: 1=highest, 3=lowest	1.540	35	1.080	36	0.001
Rank of admiration of Einstein as compared with Churchill and Freud: 1=most admired, 3=least	1.470	36	2.000	36	0.007
Number of summers spent in a research-oriented job	1.458	72	0.838	37	0.057
Rank "Doing work that involves scientific method and research" as important in being a doctor: 1=most important, 9=least	4.597	72	6.562	32	0.001

Rank importance of "Being able to deal with people rather than things", in selection of career of medicine: 1=important, 2=less, 3=little or no importance	1.423	52	1.115	26	0.030
Estimation of the percentage of time the respondent expects to spend in teaching	13.61	36	6.39	36	0.004
Estimation of the percentage of time the respondent expects to spend in patient care	65.08	36	77.53	36	0.032
Estimation of the percentage of time the respondent expects to spend in administration	7.18	55	15.74	27	0.002
Estimation of the percentage of time the respondent would like to spend in research	24.94	71	16.38	29	0.023
Estimation of the percentage of time respondent would like to spend in administration	4.41	51	13.27	26	0.001
Was any other profession besides medicine seriously considered? 1=yes, 2=no	1.444	36	1.222	36	0.047
Was teaching in college considered? 1=yes, 2=no	1.917	72	1.758	33	0.026
Was law considered? 1=yes, 2=no	1.889	72	1.576	33	0.001
Was psychology considered? 1=yes, 2=no	1.972	72	1.727	33	0.001
Was business considered? 1=yes, 2=no	1.890	36	2.000	36	0.041
Did the respondent have any doubts about becoming a doctor after decision to go to medical school had been made? 1=serious doubts, 2=slight, 3=no doubts at all	2.173	52	1.692	26	0.007
Hardest year at medical school (forecast) from first (=1) to fourth (=4)	1.493	71	1.156	32	0.027
II. Values					
Rate the importance of "being looked up to" as a factor in choice of career of medicine: 1=important, 0=not important	0.58	36	0.31	36	0.018
Rate the importance of "income and stability" as a factor in choice of career of medicine: 0=not important, 1=important	0.56	36	0.31	36	0.043
Personal feelings toward sick people who are "down and out": 1=positive feelings, 2=neutral, 3=negative	1.67	36	1.33	36	0.029

Table 4-2 continued

Matriculation Data	Careers at Graduation				
	Bioscientific Mean	N	Biosocial Mean	N	Sig
Rate importance of "being able to change society" in doctor's priorities: 1=most important, 9=least important	6.161	62	4.958	24	0.048
Rate "participation in community affairs" as an important activity after graduation from medical school: 1=highest valued activity, 6=lowest valued	4.25	36	3.72	36	0.031
Should "fee for service" be retained for the majority of physicians? 1=yes, 2=no	1.14	35	1.34	35	0.053
Should "fee for service" be retained for the respondent? 1=yes, 2=no	1.18	35	1.44	36	0.016
III. Lifestyle					
Rate "group practice with salary" as a mode of practice: 1=most favored, 2=least favored	2.67	36	2.14	35	0.008
IV. Achievement in medical school					
NBME Scores: Anatomy	555.42	72	466.62	37	0.001
Physiology	588.61	72	506.08	37	0.001
Biochemistry	618.82	72	543.12	37	0.001
Pathology	553.13	72	498.24	37	0.007
Microbiology	579.86	72	491.49	37	0.001
Pharmacology	552.92	72	510.81	37	0.024
PART I TOTAL	586.74	72	504.86	37	0.001
NBME Scores: Medicine	579.24	72	532.08	36	0.008
Surgery	547.92	72	513.06	36	0.045
Obstetrics-Gynecology	541.75	72	470.83	36	0.001
PART II TOTAL	572.92	72	536.11	36	0.048
Psychiatry	516.53	72	555.42	36	0.049

istics that were a combination of the student-practitioner and the student-psychiatrist.

The Primary Care and Increasing Governmental Control Era

Presently, we are in the Primary Care and Increasing Governmental Control Era. An examination of the data on the National Representative Sample of Medical Students at graduation, classified on the basis of whether the students choose primary care or other specialties (Table 4-3), shows that many of the major differences seen in the previous era have disappeared. What was so highly significant is either no longer significant or is a trend. In the two groups, there are no longer differences between men and women in their choice of careers, both groups are now science majors, and both derive their greatest satisfaction from the same academic subjects.

There are trends indicating that more of the students choosing nonprimary care specialties still see themselves as primarily scientists; students in the primary care group see themselves as primarily oriented toward working directly with people using science pragmatically, but in addition, show a marked interest in psychological medicine. The nonprimary care group plans to earn higher incomes. More primary care students plan to practice in deprived areas.

ANALYSES OF FINDINGS

These data clearly show that during the different eras of medicine, the characteristics of physicians who provided primary care have changed. During the Specialty Era—the days of the general practitioner—the characteristics were those of the student-practitioner who had relatively low MCAT scores, had measured interests in interpersonal relationships, wanted to work directly with people using science pragmatically, and had few intellectual interests and little interest in social factors. During the Scientific Era, students choosing primary care practically disappeared, with the vast majority of students who originally planned such careers switching to psychiatry. During the Student Activism Era, it was the student activist who saw this career as a means of changing society and effecting social change. During the Doldrums Era, the individuals choosing primary care were largely students from low income families and women who were a combination of the student-practitioner and the student-psychiatrist with a measure of social activism. During the beginning of the Primary Care and Increasing Governmental Control Era, many student-scientists (bioscientific students), in addition to the students who

Table 4–3.   National Representative Sample at Graduation 1975

	Careers at Graduation	
	Specialty Care (%)	*Primary Care (%)*
1. Basic characteristics		
Personal data		
Sex Males	51.2	48.8
Females	45.3	54.7
Geographic Origin	–	–
Parent income	Higher	Moderate
Social class	–	–
Preparation		
Undergraduate major science	82	78
Pleasure from science	–	–
Pleasure from humanities	–	–
Grades in science	–	–
Grades in nonscience	–	–
Considered other careers		
Science Ph.D.	54.2	48.2
Humanities Ph.D.	8.5	16.3
Social sciences	7.6	3.7
Psychology	14.4	14.8
Business	16.1	11.9
Teaching, elementary or high school	19.5	33.3
Law	25.4	9.6
Importance in choice of career		
Intellectual content	57.0	37.0
Social factors	16.7	37.5
Working hours	6.1	1.3
Affiliation with medical school	75.2	45.3
Source of patients		
Referred	64.5	9.5
Selected by patient	15.4	74.0
Assigned	20.2	16.5
Work in deprived area	19.9	40.7
Work beyond expectations		
Wish for advancement competetive	26.8	5.3
Patients	81.3	88.8
Doubts about Ph.D.	30.1	25.7
Plan Ph.D.	9.5	2.2
Admire Einstein, Freud, Pasteur	First in both groups	
No difference in attitudes toward patients		
No difference in amount owed		
Like about medicine		
Deal directly with people	54.9	75.4
Doing work scientifically	25.0	12.5
Excellent income	21.2	14.7

Table 4-3 continued

	Careers at Graduation	
	Specialty Care (%)	Primary Care (%)
People and research	22.0	3.0
Fee for service retained	71.5	70.7
Group practice	97.0	91.3
Allow more time with family	47.5	49.0
Plan internship in		
Specialized hospital	73.0	48.0
Community hospital	27.0	51.0
Ten years later		
Highly specialized hospital	64.0	24.0
Community hospital	36.0	76.0
Values		
Art of medicine	24.8	37.4
Competence	38.5	36.1
Delivery of care	24.8	18.5
Research	7.3	.4
Preventive aspects	8.9	7.5
Importance in career		
Intellectual	36.1	16.4
Interpersonal relationships	55.1	72.6
Introspection	9.3	11.1
Consider self		
Competetive	11.1	3.9
Equal	50.6	42.3
Cooperative	38.2	53.8
Earn money	–	–
Consider self		
Primarily scientist	40.6	20.2
Interpersonal	53.3	76.2
Psychological	6.1	3.6

combined the characteristics of student-practitioners and student-psychiatrists (biosocial students), joined the group planning primary care. This was because students perceived correctly that careers in academic and subspecialty medicine and surgery were not feasible economically.

This crossover of bioscientific students into primary care resulted in the abolition of the differences between students planning careers in primary care and those planning careers in nonprimary care specialties. Differences are only trends in the current era, whereas they had been highly significant during the Doldrums Era. This phenomenon is similar to two previous transition periods in the project when the basic characteristics of students failed to relate significantly to the career choices at graduation due to overwhelming societal factors.

The first was the transition from the Specialty to the Scientific Era when, due to the ideology and increased funding of science, a number of biosocial students elected bioscientific careers while many other biosocial students who had entered medical school planning to become general practitioners elected psychiatry. In the brief, unstable Student Activism Era, many bioscientific students, particularly at the end of their sophomore year, opted for family medicine or public health because of the ideology of the times. Within two years, these bioscientific students had reverted to bioscientific careers. These data show that in transitional periods, when ideology and funding are paramount issues, many students change their careers to those that are inappropriate to their basic characteristics. This does not occur during stable periods, as exemplified in the Specialty, Scientific, and Doldrums Eras.

Nostalgically, many would like to recall the ideal image of the kindly general practitioner and family physician of the fifties and earlier. Today, students with characteristics similar to those who went to medical school in the fifties and became general practitioners are not securing entrance to medical school, although a large number of them still apply. This raises the question of whether students with these characteristics, who typify the general practitioner of the past, should be admitted to medical school today. Our data suggest that they are not suitable for the delivery of primary care today. They lack sufficient scientific ability and knowledge as well as the public health orientation needed in such practice. In the Association of American Medical Colleges longitudinal study of the Class of 1960, one school, where the great majority of students entered general practice, had mean MCAT scores below 500.[7]

In 1973, the hypothesis was developed that the physicians graduating in the fifties who went into general practice had characteristics similar to the students currently enrolled in physicians' associate and physicians' assistant programs. The Duke program for educating physicians' associates is a good example. When this program began in the early 1960s, students were corpsmen with high school educations or less who were planning to become physicians' assistants. They would gather data, take histories, and do physicals, but would not make diagnoses. This changed, and by 1973, 50 percent of the entering class were college graduates, 37 percent had two years of college, 13 percent had some college, and all had college courses in biology and chemistry.[8]

The aim of the program was no longer to train "data gatherers" but to develop a program that would provide a basic medical curriculum.

Because of the complexities of medical practice and the changing patterns of health care delivery, it was decided not to develop a task-oriented training program. Rather, a basic medical curriculum at the undergraduate level was formulated so that graduates would possess a broad understanding of theoretical and scientific concepts. This was preferred since it would allow the graduate to continue to function effectively for ten or twenty years when current task-oriented skills would probably be outmoded. Another factor considered in this decision was that defining the role would be impossible, since every physician performs somewhat differently from every other physician.[9]

This statement could apply equally as well to physicians' education.

To test the hypothesis that students in these programs were similar to medical students who became practitioners in the 1950s, data were collected on the students in the Duke Physicians' Associate Program in 1973. Their verbal and quantitative scores on the college boards averaged 546. These scores were comparable to those of medical students entering general practice in the fifties, but far below those of medical students in 1973. On the Strong Vocational Interest Blank, these students showed a pattern of interests similar to those of the general practitioner of the 1950s but dissimilar to primary care practitioners today. The physicians' associates were interested in working directly with people, but were without measured interests in the sciences or psychology. They were concerned with the individual patient, not with social programs. They would use science pragmatically to solve problems.

Of all of the data collected, it was striking how similar the findings were for the general practitioners who graduated in the fifties and the physicians' associates of 1973. This raises an interesting question. Is the failure of many physicians to keep pace with modern advances in medicine due to the low academic ability of many of them who were admitted during the fifties and early sixties when the applicant pool was small and grades and MCAT scores were low? Reference has been made to one medical school where the MCAT score average for the class of 1960 was below 500. Many students admitted during that period also had low GPAs. Medical schools, realizing the problem, launched programs to attract more able students to medicine.

Since 1973, because of the increasing difficulty of securing entrance to medical school or finding employment commensurate with education, the qualifications of entering physicians' assistants have risen. In 1976, all students in an eastern university's physicians' assistant program are college graduates and have average college board scores in the 600s.

Most medical school admission committees favor bioscientific students over biosocial students. Early in the Doldrums Era, biosocial students at Harvard Medical School were mainly women and minority groups students. As this era developed and as the Primary Care and Increasing Governmental Control Era began, the percentage of bioscientific students among the women admitted increased. These data show that within the pool of women applicants, there were increasing numbers who entered college who planned to go to graduate school in science but changed their plans to medical school because they no longer saw science as a viable career economically. A much higher percentage of the admitted women had changed their careers during college from science to medicine than the percentage in the pool, showing the preference of the admissions committee. Many of these women preferred Ph.Ds to M.D.s and planned scientific research in a basic science while supporting themselves in primary care. This was also true for male entrants.

Because of the lack of places in academic medicine, surgery, and a number of subspecialties, many bioscientific students are being forced into primary care by economic factors. Four viewpoints prevail. Medical school faculty consider this to be a boon for medicine, and believe that the more able the student scientifically, the more able he or she will be in any field, including primary care.

Another view corresponds to the evidence that I. Berg[10] compiled in many occupations, namely, that overeducation or inappropriate education for a particular job results in poor performance and is just as detrimental as undereducation. It may well be that bioscientific students, if forced to practice in a way not related to their interests, education, aptitudes, and plans, will be disgruntled and therefore do a poor job in primary care. This is also the view of C.A. Janeway.[11]

Still another view is that these bioscientific students in primary care will adapt, change, and become competent primary care physicians. This is based on the experience in World War II of converting physicians who were not psychiatrists into psychiatrists. A large percentage remained in this specialty after leaving the service.[12]

A fourth view, expressed by E. Ginsberg,[13] is that since physicians are often not subject to all of the laws of the marketplace, they will raise their fees, overtreat, and overoperate to earn a living and not be forced into careers they do not prefer. The PSRO and similar legislation may prevent this from happening.

The data compiled on this project show that in the transitional period from the Specialty to the Scientific Era, many biosocial students changed their characteristics to bioscientific students when new opportunities arose.[14] However, they were not coerced to do so.

Medical school faculty, society, and organized medicine were in favor of the new era, and vast amounts of funds were appropriated to support it. At the time of the transition from the Scientific to the Student Activism Era, students who desired the change were opposed by the faculty and were not supported by society or financially by the government, and thus, the movement soon died. The current movement into primary care contains many students who desire this goal, but also many who would prefer other careers but who are being forced into primary care by economic necessity. There is government funding as well as support from society. It can be predicted that many will accept the inevitable, change some of their characteristics and do well in primary care; others will compromise; and probably some will be disillusioned, bitter, and become poor deliverers of primary care. This is a problem that needs to be addressed.

Chapter 5

Women in Medicine

In studying the careers of women medical students and physicians, vast quantities of data were collected and analyzed with interesting results. Women have changed markedly over the years of the project both in their career choices and in their attitudes. As a result of these changes, the career choices and attitudes of women and men currently show few differences, whereas in the past they were siginificant. To conclude that this was due to changes in women alone would be to give a false picture; men have also changed. These changes in both sexes, as well as the inter-relationship of these changes, is interesting and complex. However, in this chapter we plan only to focus on the principal changes in women, with some comparison made to the changes in men.

The major aspects of the career choices of women students include their career choices during the past twenty-eight years and changes in their backgrounds, preparation, attitudes, and a variety of other factors during the past nineteen years.

CAREER CHOICES IN THE PAST
TWENTY-EIGHT YEARS

In 1959, a booklet was published by the Harvard Medical Alumni Association describing the first decade (1948-1958) of women in the medical school.[1] From data obtained from the booklet, the career choices of the women could be determined (see Table 5-1). During the decade, 51.4 percent chose the present primary care specialties, another 25.5 percent chose psychiatry, and only 25.7 percent selected

Table 5-1.   Specialty Choices of Harvard Medical Women at Graduation

	1949-1959		
	Number of Students	*Primary Care (%)*	*Total Class (%)*
Primary care			
Vehicle			
Family (general practice)	3	3.8	4.3
General internal medicine	11	32.4	15.7
General pediatrics	20	58.8	28.5
Total in primary care	34	100	48.6
Other specialties			
Psychiatry	18 (50%)		25.7
Nonpsychiatry	18 (50%)		25.7
	1975-1976		
Primary care			
Vehicle			
Family (general practice)	2	11.1	4.4
General internal medicine	6	33.3	13.9
General pediatrics	10	55.6	23.2
Total in primary care	18	100	41.6
Other specialties			
Psychiatry	4 (12%)		9.3
Nonpsychiatry	21 (88%)		49.2

the present day bioscientific specialties. Within the primary care group, pediatrics was the career most often chosen, with 58.8 percent, compared to internal medicine with 32.4 percent. These choices reflect the basic characteristics of women entering medical school as more often biosocial than bioscientific.

During the Scientific Era of the sixties, most students choosing bioscientific careers were men. Women showed predominantly biosocial characteristics and chose general pediatrics or psychiatry as their careers. The Scientific Era was largely a male enterprise.

During the brief Student Activism Era, the career choices of women changed in that fewer chose psychiatry and more chose family medicine. But general pediatrics was still the choice of the greatest number of women. It was men who, in great numbers, changed their choices from bioscientific to biosocial careers, largely in family medicine.

In the early years of the Doldrums Era, the percentage of women choosing general pediatrics remained constant. There was, however, a marked increase in those choosing family medicine, and a further decline in those choosing psychiatry.

In 1975-1976, the percentage of graduating women from Harvard Medical School who chose primary care careers was not significantly different from men. Women still chose pediatrics as the vehicle of primary care more often than men, although the percentage difference was not as large as in the past.

At matriculation in 1975 (class of 1979), although a higher percentage of women chose primary care than men, it was not a significant difference. More women chose family medicine, and there was little difference between women and men in choosing pediatrics.

A comparison made between the career choices of women graduating from the Harvard Medical School in the decade 1949-1959 and women graduating in 1975 and 1976 shows that the percentage in primary care has not changed. The percentage within the class, or within the primary care group choosing pediatrics, is still high and unchanged: 28.5 percent of the class in the fifties, 23.2 percent in 1975-1976; 58.8 percent of the primary care group in the first instance and 55.6 percent in the latter. The dramatic change was the decline in the percentage choosing psychiatry, down from 25.7 percent to 9.3 percent, and the increase in bioscientific specialties from 25.7 percent to 49.2 percent (see Table 5-1).

In the National Representative Sample in 1975, the significant decline in the percentage of women choosing pediatrics at matriculation paralleled the same decline in the Harvard Medical School. At matriculation in 1975, both nationally and in the Harvard Medical School, there was a marked increase in women as compared with men who chose obstetrics-gynecology (see Table 5-2). Over the years these changes have occurred in women with some concomitant changes in the career choices of men. At graduation in 1975-1976, there was no significant difference in career choices between men and women.

BACKGROUNDS AND ATTITUDES OF WOMEN: 1958-1976

There have been marked changes over the past nineteen years in the backgrounds and attitudes of women medical students and physicians per se. As imperfect as it may be, the following method has been devised to present these data.[2] Plusses and minuses are used to show the differences on selected variables. The greater the number of

Table 5-2. National Representative Sample

	Graduation 1975				Matriculation 1975			
	Men *N = 387*		*Women* *N = 84*		*Men* *N = 925*		*Women* *N = 320*	
	N	*%*	*N*	*%*	*N*	*%*	*N*	*%*
Primary care sub-divisions								
General family practice	72 = 18.6		6 = 7.2		225 = 24.5		76 = 23.8	
General internal medicine	72 = 18.6		15 = 17.9		177 = 19.3		54 = 16.9	
General pediatrics	29 = 7.5		20 = 23.8		85 = 9.3		44 = 13.6	
Total in primary care	173 = 44.7		41 = 48.8		487 = 53.1		174 = 54.4	
Other specialties	214 = 55.3		43 = 51.2		438 = 47.8		146 = 45.6	
Obstetrics-Gynecology	16 = 4.1		5 = 6.0		9 = 1.0		31 = 9.7	
Psychiatry	12 = 3.1		8 = 9.5		16 = 1.7		10 = 3.0	
Other	186 = 48.8		30 = 35.7		413 = 45.0		105 = 32.8	

plusses, the larger the number of students who answered the question the same; the greater the difference in the number of plusses, the greater the difference between the subjects on a particular variable. Minuses are used when a very small number of students answered the question in that direction. These data are shown in Table 5-3, which compares men with women at three periods: Harvard medical alumni-alumnae in the classes from 1958 to 1972 using data collected in 1975; a national sample of medical students at graduation (class of 1975); and a sample at matriculation in 1975 (class of 1979).

RESULTS

In general, the results show that on many variables, women have changed in their backgrounds, career plans, and attitudes as compared with men. They have moved closer to men on most variables, although on a few differences still exist.

For example, in terms of background, women physicians who graduated from medical school prior to 1975 came from families of a higher social class than males, from families where a much greater number of their mothers had careers, and from families where their mothers had more education than males. However, for women entering medical school in 1975, there were no differences on any of these variables.

Table 5-3.   Women Medical Students and Physicians as Compared with Men Medical Students and Physicians

	National Sample 1975 Matriculation	National Sample 1975 Graduation	Harvard Medical School Alumnae 1975
1. Social class	–	Upper	Upper
2. Geographic origin	–	–	–
3. Career mother	–	++++	++++
4. Year's of mother's education	–	++++	++++
5. Pleasure from science	+	+	+
Pleasure from humanities	+++	+++	+++
6. Highest grades	–	Humanities	Humanities
Alternate career	–	Public health	Ph.D. humanities
			School teacher
			Social work
7. Medical career	All careers	General specialty	General specialty
		Psychiatry	Psychiatry
		Public Health	
8. Hours of work	Less than men (10 hours)	Less than men (10 hours)	Less than men (10 hours)
9. Income	Less than men	Less than men	Less than men
10. Effect of social factors on career	–	–	++++
11. Family practice vehicle	++	+++	+++
Medicine	+++	++	++
General family medicine	+++	+	–
12. Consider Self			
Primarily scientist	+	+	+
Primarily interpersonal	+++	+++	+++
Competetive	++	+	+
Cooperative	++	+++	+++
13. Family practitioner	–	–	–
14. Deprived area	–	–	–

Table 5-3 continued

	National Sample 1975 Matriculation	National Sample 1975 Graduation	Harvard Medical School Alumnae 1975
15. Primary care	-	-	+++
16. Like about medicine			
People	+++	+++	+++
Psychological problems	++	++	++
Change society	++	++	-
17. If in deprived area			
Ghetto	+	+	+++
Rural	+++	+++	+
18. Values			
Art of medicine	-	-	-
19. Competence	-	-	-
Delivery of care	-	-	-
Research	-	-	-
Prevention			-
19. Favor abolishing			
fee for service	+++	+++	+

Key: Plusses and minuses are used to show the differences on selected variables. The greater the number of plusses, the larger the number of students who answered the question the same; the greater the difference in the number of plusses, the greater the difference between the subjects on a particular variable. Minuses are used when a very small number of students answered the question in that direction.

For the alumnae group and for women graduating from medical school in 1975 who had matriculated in 1971, their highest college grades were in the humanities, whereas males made their highest college grades in the sciences. However, for women entering medical school in 1975, grades in science and in the humanities did not differ from those of men. All three groups of women reported that their greatest satisfaction academically came from the study of the humanities and not from science. This did not change over the years.

The alternate careers considered by men and women before entering medical school differed markedly in the alumni-alumnae and in the graduating class of 1975. In the group graduating prior to 1972, women had considered a Ph.D. in humanities, school teaching, and social work, whereas men in this group had considered business, law, and engineering. For the class graduating in 1975, women had considered a Ph.D. in the humanities, and a sizable number had considered public health; men had considered law and engineering. But for the class entering in 1975, there were no differences in the alternate careers considered by men and women, with both now considering the range of careers including Ph.D.s in science, law, business, and engineering.

In geographic location, there were no differences in the percentage of women and men planning to practice or practicing in deprived areas in all three groups. However, in the alumni-alumnae group, for those practicing in a medically deprived area, the majority of women were in slums, while men practiced in rural areas. For the groups graduating or matriculating in 1975, increasing numbers were planning to practice in medically underserviced areas, but both men and women planned to make their careers in rural rather than slum areas.

On two variables related to careers, the same differences between men and women were found in all three groups. Women worked and planned to work an average of ten hours less than men, and their incomes or planned incomes were considerably lower than those of men.

On the effects of social factors on their careers, women who graduated prior to 1973 saw social factors as a marked obstacle to their careers. Family responsibilities were infrequently mentioned, while the prejudice of men in medicine against women was most often cited. Some women felt that having a husband to support them contributed to their career, giving them the freedom to make career choices without regard to finances. A number of men stated that family financial obligations played a significant role in their careers. They frequently worked long hours for extra funds, or made less fulfilling career choices, choosing positions that enabled them to earn more money. Thus the same percentage of men as women saw family obligations as interfering with their career, but in different ways. The prejudice of male physicians against women in medicine was seen by almost all of the women as the great obstacle; a majority of the men saw this prejudice against women as the greatest problem faced by women.

For students graduating or matriculating in 1975, there were no differences between men and women in the percentage who thought social factors would be a problem in their careers. Women no longer felt that men were prejudiced against them.

In all three groups, women saw themselves primarily interested in interpersonal relationships whereas men saw themselves primarily interested in science. Both the women who graduated prior to 1973 and those who graduated in 1975 saw themselves as far less competitive and more cooperative than men. However, with the class entering in 1975, this has changed. Women see themselves equally as competitive and cooperative as men.

SUMMARY

These data show clearly that over the years women medical students and physicians have changed in their backgrounds, careers, and attitudes. Men have also changed, and these changes, combined with those by women, have erased many of the differences between men and women so prevalent in the past. For example, formerly, most women medical students came from a high social class where mothers had careers and were better educated, whereas today this differential, compared with men, no longer exists. In the past, if women had not secured entrance to medical school, they considered alternate careers in more traditional fields open to women such as school teaching or social work, whereas today they choose the same alternates as men— Ph.D.s in science, careers in business or law, and the like.

In the past, women specialized principally in psychiatry or primary care, usually pediatrics, whereas today there is little difference between the careers planned by entering female and male medical students, except for slightly more women in obstetrics-gynecology. In the past, women who planned careers in deprived areas were apt to work in slums, males in rural areas. Today both groups plan to work in rural areas.

Women in the past felt that social factors, which they identified as the prejudice against them by male physicians, impeded their progress. Today's medical students think that this is no longer a factor.

In the past, women saw themselves as far more cooperative and much less competitive than men. Today's women medical students feel that they are just as competitive as men.

Some variables have not changed. Women in college still derive their greatest satisfaction from studying the humanities. In science, their grades are equal to men's, although in the past they were not. Women do not work or plan to work as many hours a week as men, nor do they make or plan to make as much money.

The changes in women reflect the changes in society's attitudes toward women and of women toward society. Additionally, they are partially related to the applicant pool and the admission policies of medical schools. These data show that few women admitted prior to 1973 considered a Ph.D. in science, although many men did. However, today a good number of women admitted to medical school had planned to get Ph.D.s in science when they entered college, but changed their careers to medicine because they felt that the prospects for scientists were bleak. With increasing numbers of such women in the applicant pool, medical schools will choose the more scientifically oriented women in greater numbers.

This raises the much debated question: Do women bring something special to medicine that men do not? Do their special traits encompass more consideration for children, the psychological aspects of illness, the emotional component of medicine, and the more humanistic aspects of care? Examples of the different attitudes among Harvard medical alumnae include, on one hand, the woman who became a professor of surgery and felt that at last she had reached a position where she is professionally equal. She is no longer known as a "lady surgeon" but as "a surgeon." The other attitude is exemplified by the woman pediatrician who developed an outstanding pediatric clinic in the slums. She believed that no one but a woman could have done this, and that it is a unique contribution of women.[3] This is, in fact, a moot question. Because of the increasing number of scientifically oriented women being admitted to medical school, the real question is: Will today's women medical students revert to the more traditional roles of women in medicine after graduation or will they assume the same roles as men? Only followup studies will determine this.

The oldest women studied in this project were seventeen years out of medical school, with an average age of forty-three at the time of the followup studies in 1975. These worked an average of ten hours less per week than men. If these same facts remain until they are fifty-one when their family obligations will have been fulfilled, the average woman will have worked approximately two years less than the average man. These facts do not reveal whether or not women contribute as much as men in hours worked. This can only be determined by studying a group of women over their entire lifetime. Due to the increased longevity of women over men, especially late in life, a projection of these data may well show that women work more work years than men. Another factor that must be considered in assessing this difference in amount of work is the changing lifestyle of young women who are increasing their time in work commitments away from their homes.

Women make or plan to make less money than men. This could be related to their shorter work week, to being paid less than men for the same position, or to taking positions that are low paying because of their social connotations. More intensive studies are needed in this area.

Another interesting point was the attitudes of women about social factors as obstacles to their medical careers. The majority of alumnae felt that their careers had been difficult because of prejudice from male physicians. Surprisingly, only a small percentage mentioned family obligations as interfering with their careers. These attitudes no longer prevail. Among both senior women medical students and those matriculating in 1975, only a small percentage felt that social factors would impede their progress. An equally small percentage of men medical students in these two groups felt that prejudice in favor of women or minorities might impede their careers.

In the alumni sample, a significant number of males felt that being the sole support of their families had impeded their careers because they had to make choices that were financially rather than career based. In the alumnae sample, a significant number of women felt that their marriages had helped their careers because a second income allowed them to choose the course that would advance their careers without regard to finances.

Changes took place over the years, and today there are almost no differences in the career choices of women and men. The similarities in their backgrounds and attitudes is a result of the significant changes in both men and women regarding their career choices in recent years.

❋ *Chapter 6*

Current Issues in Medicine

The data collected on the National Sample of Medical Students at graduation and matriculation in 1975 shed light on a number of important current issues. Several pieces of federal legislation address these issues and are expected to have profound implications for medicine.

First is the Professional Standards Review Organization (PSRO) that seeks to insure the quality of medical care. Also looming on the horizon are state laws for relicensing and specialty board requirements for recertification. Second is the passage of the Manpower Act in 1976, which seeks to control the specialty choice of graduating students and to create a geographical redistribution. This act will force students who go into the National Health Service Corps to become primary care physicians in underserviced areas in order to finance their educations. They will give one year of service for each year of educational aid. The third piece of pending legislation is national health insurance, although it is not possible at this time to predict when or in what form it will be passed.

Undoubtedly, these measures will have a profound impact on the redistribution of physicians within specialties as well as geographically. If the PSRO mechanism works, one effect will be the redistribution of physicians. Many economists have pointed out that physians make their own market by overoperating and overtreating. Strict quality standards would diminish this practice, thus forcing many physicians to move from overserviced areas, such as the suburbs, to less serviced areas such as slums and rural areas.

ECONOMIC FACTORS AND
CAREER CHOICE

It is ironic that at the very time that legislation is passed to redistribute physicians, there are indications that the economics of supply and demand are forcing changes in specialization and geographic distribution. For example, at this time there are too many general surgeons, and many young physicians in that specialty are forced to become emergency room physicians or to go into other types of practice. Due to the lack of funding, many physicians who would prefer and who are educated for full-time academic careers—principally in research or teaching, with some patient care—are being forced into practice with or without a part-time medical school affiliation. In some medical subspecialties, because of excess numbers, many are practicing general internal medicine with special attention to their subspecialty. Again, these physicians would prefer to devote full-time to their subspecialties. Moreover, data show that many students are planning careers different from their preferred careers. This is most marked among those preferring careers in surgery or in academic medicine who are now planning alternative careers.

Another factor that is affecting medical practice is the declining birth rate. Many general pediatricians are having difficulty securing patients. This is especially true in the suburbs where, in some cases, elementary schools are being closed for lack of children. The makers of Gerber® baby foods have been forced to diversify and to close some of their plants. Increasing numbers of faimly physicians will take children away from pediatricians. Undoubtedly, some pediatricians will have to move to underserviced areas or be retrained as family physicians.

CHANGES IN THE CAREER CHOICES
OF PHYSICIANS

It is now evident that many more graduates than in the recent past will have careers in primary medicine—general internal medicine, general pediatrics, and general family practice—because of economic factors, the demands of society, and federal and state legislation. Already, it is apparent that there is an oversupply of surgeons, medical subspecialists, diagnostic radiologists, and academicians. Many young physicians trained in these specialties are having to move into other specialties or, most frequently, are being forced to include a large component of primary care in their practice. The mechanisms now being developed to insure the competence of physicians, thus preventing overtreatment and overoperating, may also expedite the change. The Robert Wood Johnson Foundation, by focusing on this problem and making primary care opportunities available, has been the major catalyst in this change in the career plans of many students and young physicians.

The data collected in this study show that in the past, as each new era approached, the harbingers of the new era occurred in the student body in increasing numbers. Table 2-2 shows the number of seniors in 1975 planning careers in primary care. The data on the National Intern and Resident Matching Program in 1977 was summarized by Cooper as follows:

> This year's matching confirms a strong move toward students entering careers in primary care specialties (family medicine, internal medicine and pediatrics), which represents a four year trend. There will be 7,590 students entering residency programs in the designated primary care specialties. This is 2,263 more than entered these specialties in 1974 and represents a 42 percent increase in the four years. . . .
>
> Of all the students who were matched (12,760), sixty percent chose the designated primary care specialties and 16 percent will enter surgery and the surgical subspecialties. Of the remaining 3,062 students, fifteen percent will begin training for careers in specialties such as obstetrics, radiology, anesthesiology, pathology and physical medicine while eight percent have opted for general first-year programs, planning to decide on their areas of specialization the following year.
>
> The AAMC is encouraged by the growing interest in primary care evidenced by the matching program results for the class of 1977. The expanding number of U.S. medical graduates and the increasing proportion entering the primary care specialties confirms the clear response of the Nation's medical schools to the need for more physicians who will provide primary medical services.[1]

This raises the question of how long it will take to oversaturate the market with primary care physicians. As mentioned, due to the falling birth rate, many suburban pediatricians are having difficulty securing patients. In interviews with them they attack pediatric nurse practitioners, whom they feel are taking patients away from them. Many pediatricians are considering retraining as family practitioners rather than moving to underserviced areas. Soon 15,000 physicians will be graduated each year. If such a high percentage continues to choose primary care, one result may be the displacement of physician assistants and nurse practitioners in primary care. The reverse effect can be seen in surgery, where many physician assistants are being employed by hospitals to do the work formerly done by interns. These hospitals are unable to secure interns due to the decreased numbers of medical students choosing that specialty.

METHOD OF PRACTICE

These data, as well as those of others such as the California Medical Association,[2] show that the overwhelming majority of medical students and young physicians plan to practice in groups (see Table 6-1). They see this as enabling them to work fewer hours, thus making it possible to spend more time with their families and to engage in other activities (see Table 6-2). The need for physicians, however, may increase if physicians start working fewer hours. (See Table 6-3.)

What will be the principal vehicle for the delivery of primary care? The data show that it may not be general family practice. Table 2-3 shows that general internal medicine and general pediatrics together exceed general family practice as the choice of those planning careers in primary care. However, because of the previously mentioned difficulties faced by pediatricians, it is becoming more probable that they will secure additional training and become family practitioners.

Table 6-1. Attitudes and Values Toward Medicine of Medical Students in a National Representative Sample of Medical Schools at Graduation and Matriculation

	Graduation June 1975 Class of 1975		Matriculation September 1975 Class of 1979	
	N	*%*	*N*	*%*
1. In favor of group practice	441 =	98.8	1061 =	90.8
2. For abolishing fee for service	137 =	29.6	322 =	27.2
3. Most important values				
A. The art of medicine	142 =	30.9	331 =	28.1
B. Competence of the physician	171 =	37.2	397 =	33.7
C. Delivery of optimal care to the entire population	100 =	21.7	289 =	24.5
D. Research	8 =	1.7	32 =	2.7
E. Preventive medicine	39 =	8.5	129 =	11.0
4. Favor national health insurance	283 =	61.5	768 =	64.6
5. Plan to be politically active on matters of health	275 =	58.5	784 =	64.6
6. Like to work on a full-time basis for the government	41 =	8.9	103 =	8.5

Table 6-2. Mean Percentage of Importance for Choice of Group Practice of Medical Students in a National Representative Sample of Medical Schools in 1975 at Graduation and Matriculation

Factor	Graduation June 1975 Class of 1975 N = %	Matriculation September 1975 Class of 1979 N = %
Group enables physician to control hours of work to allow for more time with family and other outside activities	230 = 48.1	453 = 36.5
Group increases level of competence due to involvement of diverse physicians	153 = 31.9	517 = 41.6
Group allows pooling of office, lab expenses, making room for extra equipment, personnel, *etc.*	96 = 20.1	273 = 22.0

Table 6-3. Expected Working Hours per Week of Medical Students in a National Representative Sample of Medical Schools in 1975 at Graduation and Matriculation

Hours expected to work	Graduation June 1975 Class of 1975 N	%	Matriculation September 1975 Class of 1979 N	%
20–30 hours	10 =	2.1	19 =	1.6
31–40 hours	35 =	7.5	150 =	12.3
41–50 hours	157 =	33.6	476 =	39.1
51–60 hours	180 =	38.5	452 =	37.1
More than 60 hours	86 =	18.4	122 =	10.0

The economic pressures forcing many medical subspecialists to give the majority of their time to primary care can only accelerate practice in the direction of specialists in groups rather than as general family practitioners. Some of these will be multipurpose groups with lawyers, educators, social workers, and welfare officials as part of the group in which physicians work.

REDISTRIBUTION OF PHYSICIANS GEOGRAPHICALLY

Undoubtedly, the new government legislation, economic factors, and the declining birth rate will force physicians into underserviced areas. The data collected on this project (Table 6-4) show that 30.1 percent of seniors and 34.4 percent of matriculating students plan careers in underserviced areas, but that most of these students prefer rural areas. The inner city is the choice of 3.7 percent of the graduates and 5.1 percent of the matriculating students. In other words, of the total number of students electing to practice in deprived areas, 87 percent of the seniors and 82 percent of the freshmen prefer rural areas. The figures for slum areas are 12 percent and 15 percent respectively (see Table 6-5).

This movement into rural areas is not unique for physicians. In 1976, according to the U.S. Census Bureau, more people moved from cities to rural areas than vice versa for the first time. The problem now is to force physicians into ghetto areas, which will

Table 6-4. Projected Location of Practice of Medical Students in a National Representative Sample of Medical Schools in 1975 at Graduation and Matriculation

	Graduation June 1975 Class of 1975		Matriculation September 1975 Class of 1979	
	N	%	N	%
Location:				
Slums	17 =	3.7	61 =	5.1
Rural area	121 =	26.2	336 =	28.1
Indian reservation	1 =	0.2	14 =	1.2
Total in *Deprived area:*	139 =	30.1	411 =	34.4
Suburbs	176 =	38.1	399 =	33.4
Urban: nonghetto area	132 =	28.6	328 =	27.5
Foreign country	10 =	2.2	40 =	3.4
Military service	5 =	1.1	16 =	1.3
Total in *Nondeprived area:*	323* =	70.0	783 =	65.6
Grand totals:	462* = 100		1194** = 100	
Mean time expected in:				
Deprived area:		33.3		37.2
Nondeprived area:		66.7		62.8

*Seventeen out of 479 respondents failed to specify a practice location.
**Forty-eight out of 1,242 respondents failed to specify a practice location.

Table 6-5. The Percentage of Students in the National Representative Sample Planning Practice in Deprived Areas

	Graduation 1975		Matriculation 1975	
	N	%	N	%
Slums	17 =	12	61 =	15
Rural area	121 =	87	336 =	82
Indian reservation	1 =	01	14 =	03
Total in deprived areas	139 =	100	411 =	100

undoubtedly require government action. According to our data, there is no evidence that this would be done voluntarily.

DEPRIVED AREAS

The need for a redistribution of physicians into medically deprived areas, slums, and rural areas has a high national priority. Many efforts have been made in the past to attract physicians to rural areas without much success. The National Health Service Corps, which was expanded by the Manpower Act of 1976, may change this.

The National Sample of Medical Students studied in this project in 1975 shows that 30.1 percent of those graduating and 34.4 percent of those matriculating plan to practice in a medically deprived area. Only 3.7 percent at graduation and 5.1 percent at matriculation plan to practice in slum areas. In contrast, 26.2 percent and 28.1 percent respectively plan to practice in rural areas (see Table 6-4). If we look at the total number planning to practice in a deprived area, 87 percent of those graduating and 81.1 percent of those matriculating choose rural areas. The movement toward slums is small; 12.1 percent at graduation and 14.8 percent at matriculation (see Table 6-5). The students planning practice in a deprived area use the vehicle of general family practice rather than general internal medicine or general pediatrics (see Table 6-6).

The characteristics of students planning practice in deprived areas may be seen in Table 6-7 and can be categorized as follows. They come significantly from rural areas and less affluent families. They do not place a high value on status or financial rewards. Evidence for their lack of emphasis on status and prestige are their alternate careers, which are most frequently high school or elementary teaching and social work. Students in primary care not planning to work in deprived areas frequently have a Ph.D. in science or other high status occupations as alternate careers.

Table 6-6. Primary Care Vehicle and Practice Location of Medical Students Planning Primary Care Practice in a National Representative Sample of Medical Schools at Graduation in 1975

Primary Care	Practice Location	
	Deprived Areas	*Nondeprived Areas*
Vehicle	*(N = 137)* N %	*(N = 306)* N %
General internal medicine and general pediatrics	62 = 13	233 = 53
Family practice	75 = 17	73 = 17

Chi square = 21.58 with one degree of freedom significance <.01.

These students are socially more concerned. This is shown by their plans to be politically more active and to advocate prepayment practice. They see medicine as a vehicle to change society. They have a preventive medicine outlook and are postively related to patients with psychological problems, the elderly, and the worried well—all seen negatively by primary care physicians not in deprived areas. They do not see themselves as scientists, but are primarily people-oriented and cooperative rather than competitive.

In summary, these students come from rural areas; place little emphasis on prestige, status, and financial rewards; are much more politically active; are less conservative; have a public health orientation and emphasize working with people in a cooperative way; are intensely interested in the psychological problems of patients; and are also interested in working with the aged. They plan general family practice. This is a unique cluster of characteristics. Although many of these students have characteristics in common with those who plan to practice primary care, regardless of geographic location, their characteristics are more marked.

Two other important considerations are the relationship between the place where a student is reared and the place of practice, and the relationship of social class of the student's father to the place of practice. Tables 6-8 and 6-9 show that a significantly larger number of students at matriculation and graduation than would be expected by chance, who come from rural areas, plan to practice in a rural area. At matriculation, twenty-nine or 50 percent of the students planning to practice in a slum area are from large cities; a further analysis of these data show that most of them come from slum areas.

Table 6-7. National Sample of Medical Students at Matriculation and Graduation in 1975: Alumni-Alumnae of Harvard Medical School in 1975

	Specialty Practice	Primary Care	Deprived Area
1. Social class	–	–	–
2. Geographic origin	–	–	Rural or small town
3. Major in college	–		–
4. Reason for career	Intellectual	Social	Social
5. Alternate career:	Ph.D. Science	High school or ele-mentary teaching	High school or elementary teaching
	Law	Ph.D. Science	Social Work
	Engineering		Public Health
6. Income	Very high	High	Moderate
7. Source of income	Employment	Fee for service	Prepayment
8. Like about medicine			
Colleagues	++++	++	–
Income	++++	++	–
Research	++++	++	–
Patient care	++	+++	++++
Change society	–	+	+++
Prevention	–	–	+++
9. Attitudes toward patients			
Psychological problems	+	+	++++
Old people	+	+	++++
Worried well	+	+	++++
10. Consider self primarily			
Scientist	+++	++	–
Work with people	+	+++	++++
Competitive	+++	++	–
Cooperative	+	++	++++
11. Practice	Subspecialty	General specialty	General family medicine

Table 6–7 continued

	Specialty Practice	Primary Care	Deprived Area
12. Values			
Art of medicine	–	+++	+++
Competence	+++	+++	++
Delivery of care	+	++	+++
Research	++	–	–
Prevention	–	–	++
13. Sex	–	Women alumnae	–
14. Politically active	++	++	++++

Key: Plusses and minuses are used to show the differences on selected variables. The greater the number of plusses, the larger the number of students who answered the question the same; the greater the difference in the number of plusses, the greater the difference between the subjects on a particular variable. Minuses are used when a very small number of students answered the question in that direction.

Table 6-8. Home Towns and Practice Locations of Medical Students in a National Representative Sample of Medical Schools at Matriculation in 1975

Practice Location	Home Town													
	Farm or Ranch		Town		Small City		Suburb		Large City		Moved Around		Total	
	N	%	N	%	N	%	N	%	N	%	N	%	N	%
Slums	0 =	0	4 =	3.1	9 =	3.4	13 =	3.3	29 =	11.2	3 =	4.6	58 =	4.9
Rural	38 =	65.5	67 =	51.9	73 =	27.7	84 =	21.1	49 =	18.8	23 =	35.4	334 =	28.4
Suburbs	8 =	13.8	40 =	31.0	111 =	42.0	172 =	43.2	45 =	17.3	15 =	23.1	391 =	33.3
Urban	9 =	15.5	14 =	10.9	59 =	22.3	105 =	26.4	124 =	47.7	11 =	16.9	322 =	27.4
Foreign	0 =	0	2 =	1.6	4 =	1.5	16 =	4.0	11 =	4.2	7 =	10.8	40 =	3.4
Reservation	1 =	1.7	-		7 =	2.7	3 =	0.8	1 =	0.4	2 =	3.1	14 =	1.2
Military	2 =	3.4	2 =	1.6	1 =	0.4	5 =	1.3	1 =	0.4	4 =	6.2	15 =	1.3
Totals	58 =	100	129 =	100	264 =	100	398 =	100	260 =	100	65 =	100	1174 =	100

Chi square = 249.845. Significance under 0.001 with 30 degrees of freedom.

Table 6-9.   Home Towns and Practice Locations of Medical Students in a National Representative Sample of Medical Schools at Graduation in 1975

| | | | | | | | | | | Home Towns | | | | | | | |
Practice Location	Farm or Ranch N	%	Town N	%	Small City N	%	Suburb N	%	Large City N	%	Moved Around N	%	Total N	%
Slums	1 =	3.8	2 =	3.4	2 =	2.4	1 =	1.1	2 =	3.5	–	–	8 =	2.3
Rural	14 =	53.8	25 =	42.4	22 =	25.9	27 =	28.7	6 =	10.5	7 =	35.0	101 =	29.6
Suburbs	7 =	26.9	25 =	42.4	42 =	49.4	46 =	48.9	24 =	42.1	9 =	45.0	153 =	44.9
Urban	3 =	11.5	6 =	10.2	16 =	18.8	18 =	19.1	23 =	40.4	2 =	10.0	68 =	19.9
Foreign	1 =	3.8	1 =	1.7	1 =	1.2	1 =	1.1	1 =	1.8	1 =	5.0	6 =	1.8
Reservation	–	–	–	–	–	–	–	–	–	–	–	–	0 =	0.0
Military	–	–	–	–	2 =	2.4	1 =	1.1	1 =	1.8	1 =	5.0	5 =	1.5
Totals	26 = 100		59 = 100		85 = 100		94 = 100		57 = 100		20 = 100		341 = 100	

Chi square – 43.320. Significance at 0.014 with 25 degrees of freedom.

This, too, is statistically significant. At graduation, only eight planned to practice in a slum area, and the relationship between being raised in a large city and practicing in the slums is no longer significant. However, these data are drawn from different classes in the same year, 1975, and the number planning to practice in slums is so small that it is difficult to draw conclusions about seniors.

Tables 6-10 and 6-11 show data on the relationship of the fathers' social class and the place of practice of medical students. At matriculation, this table shows a significant relationship of place of practice to the fathers' social class. Particularly striking is the high percentage of lower social class students who plan to practice in rural areas. At graduation, this relationship no longer holds. There was no relationship between social class and planning to practice in slums at either matriculation or graduation, although the numbers planning such a practice are so small that no general conclusions should be drawn.

It is highly probable statistically that students from rural areas plan to practice in rural areas. Due to the increasing numbers in all social classes planning to practice in rural areas, it would be important to study the type of rural area in which the practice is planned—deprived areas such as Appalachia or nondeprived rural areas.

ASSURING THE COMPETENCE OF PHYSICIANS

While legislation aimed at insuring the competence of physicians and hopefully keeping down the costs of medical care has been passed, the method for insuring such competence has not yet been decided. Some possibilities are the PSROs, either alone or in combination with other methods; periodic reexamination; required continuing education; or review of physicians' records by personnel other than physicians. These data show that a majority of medical students are in favor of all of these mechanisms for insuring the competence of physicians (see Table 6-12).

THE "WORRIED WELL"

Garfield[3] stated that approximately 50 percent of patients seen by the Kaiser Permanente Group are the "worried well." These are patients who, after adequate medical workups, show no biological reason for their complaints. They are costly and time consuming for physicians, but even more important is the fact that they are seldom helped by current medical practices. Would further education of physicians in caring for the emotional problems of patients by the

Table 6–10.   Practice Location and Father's Social Class of Medical Students in a National Representative Sample of Medical Schools at Matriculation in 1975

First Choice Practice Location	I N	%	II N	%	III N	%	IV N	%	V N	%	Total N	%
							Father's Social Class					
Slums	16 =	2.9	15 =	4.8	18 =	10.6	6 =	5.5	3 =	8.8	58 =	4.9
Rural	159 =	29.1	89 =	28.4	40 =	23.5	32 =	29.1	14 =	41.2	334 =	28.4
Suburbs	186 =	34.0	111 =	35.5	51 =	30.0	35 =	31.8	8 =	23.5	391 =	33.3
Urban	151 =	27.6	79 =	25.2	51 =	30.0	31 =	28.2	9 =	26.5	321 =	27.3
Foreign	25 =	4.6	10 =	3.2	4 =	2.4	1 =	0.9	– –		40 =	3.4
Reservation	5 =	0.9	3 =	1.0	2 =	1.2	4 =	3.7	– –		14 =	1.2
Military	5 =	0.9	6 =	1.9	4 =	2.4	1 =	0.9	– –		16 =	1.4
Totals	547 =	100	313 =	100	170 =	100	110 =	100	34 =	100	1174 =	100
Deprived	180 =	32.9	107 =	34.2	60 =	35.3	42 =	38.3	17 =	50.0		
Nondeprived	367 =	67.1	206 =	65.0	110 =	64.7	68 =	61.7	17 =	50.0		

Chi square = 38.896. Significant at 0.030 with 24 degrees of freedom.

Table 6-11. Practice Location and Father's Social Class of Medical Students in a National Representative Sample of Medical Schools at Graduation in 1975

First Choice Practice Location	Father's Social Class												
	I N	%	II N	%	III N	%	IV N	%	V N	%	Total N	%
Slums	2 =	1.5	3 =	3.0	–	– –	2 =	8.7	1 =	11.1	8 =	2.3
Rural	40 =	30.5	22 =	21.8	24 =	31.2	11 =	47.8	3 =	33.3	100 =	29.3
Suburbs	57 =	43.5	52 =	51.5	37 =	48.1	6 =	26.1	2 =	22.2	154 =	45.2
Urban	27 =	20.6	21 =	20.8	13 =	16.9	4 =	17.4	3 =	33.3	68 =	19.9
Foreign	4 =	3.1	1 =	1.0	1 =	1.3	–	– –	–	– –	6 =	1.8
Reservation	–	– –	–	– –	–	– –	–	– –	–	– –	0 =	0.0
Military	1 =	0.8	2 =	2.0	2 =	2.6	–	– –	–	– –	5 =	1.5
Total	131 =	100	101 =	100	77 =	100	23 =	100	9 =	100	341 =	100

Chi square = 23.432 Significant at 0.270 with 20 degrees of freedom.

Table 6-12. Attitudes of Medical Students in a National Representative Sample of Medical Schools in 1975 at Graduation and Matriculation

	Graduation June 1975 Class of 1975		Matriculation September 1975 Class of 1975	
	N	%	N	%
In favor of states requiring relicensure every six years	324	= 68.8	909	= 74.6

answer? Or should such patients be referred to psychiatrists or be seen by professional mental health workers or allied health personnel? This is an important issue that needs discussion and research. The data that were collected show that few students are interested in this type of patient (see Table 6-13).

DEHUMANIZATION OF MEDICINE

Another issue that is receiving widespread attention is the dehumanization of medicine. As pointed out by Elliot Richardson[4] and David Rogers,[5] the dehumanization of the patient and the physician, which can only accelerate under national health insurance unless countermeasures are taken, is a vital concern. Richardson argued:

Table 6-13. Reactions of Medical Students in a National Representative Sample of Medical Schools in 1975 at Graduation and Matriculation

	Graduation June 1975 Class of 1975		Matriculation September 1975 Class of 1979	
	N	%	N	%
Reactions toward people with psychogenic symptoms:				
Negative	186	= 39.7	237	= 19.6
Neutral	193	= 41.2	644	= 53.2
Positive	89	= 19.0	330	= 27.3
Reactions toward people who have clear-cut physical illnesses:				
Negative	1	= 0.2	10	= 0.8
Neutral	99	= 21.2	367	= 30.1
Positive	368	= 78.6	844	= 69.1

Given that the federal government is increasingly to be involved in health and given that pressures toward greater "efficiency" are likely to occur, how can we prevent the alienation of the public from one more set of precious institutions? . . . Can we preserve a place of dignity and individuality for people in their relations with that system? . . . Can we prevent the undesirable depersonalization and centralization of a system that has heretofore—in spite of its criticism—been appreciated more than most for its personal and immediate characteristics? This issue or set of issues, introduces a theme that is central to what I take to be a profoundly important developing drama—a test of whether our health system or any social-service system, so beset by dehumanizing forces can long preserve its humanism—whether the best of its humanistic traditions can long endure.[6]

Can this be handled by changing institutional arrangements, or does the fault lie in the type of student being admitted to medical school, in the nature of medical education itself, or in our technological society? These data show that the issue of dehumanization is of great importance to most biosocial students, of less interest to bioscientific students. Regardless, it is an important issue for debate and research (see Table 6–14).

Table 6–14. Attitudes of Medical Students in a National Representative Sample of Medical Schools at Matriculation and Graduation in 1975

	Graduation June 1975 Class of 1975		Matriculation September 1975 Class of 1975	
	N (479)	% (100%)	N (1.242)	% (100%)
1. Depersonalization is a primary issue in patient care today.	324 =	67.6	870 =	70.0
2. Medical schools should have two different curricula: one bioscientific, the other biosocial.	129 =	26.9	422 =	33.9
3. Favor action without careful analysis first in securing changes in delivery of medical care to the community	92 =	19.2	172 =	13.8

GERIATRICS AND REHABILITATION

A major issue for medicine is the increasing numbers of the elderly. Society and physicians simply do not provide adequately for their medical care and other needs. Table 6-15 shows the attitudes of students toward children, young people, and the old as patients. Ten years ago, far more than half of the students had negative reactions toward the old; now about 45 percent have positive attitudes. How much of this is attributable to our youth-oriented society or to the nature of medical education is not known. Medical students are interested in acute illnesses of the young. Changing these attitudes is a problem for medical education.

RESEARCH

It is essential that the issues about research be resolved in favor of a balanced program of basic science and clinical research, including an evaluation of health care delivery. If research is not adequately funded, physicians in the year 2000 will be practicing 1975 medicine. Bioscientific students show interest in research but are concerned that, due to funding, they may be able to do little themselves; biosocial students show little interest in this area. The changes in attitudes toward research may be seen in Tables 2-1 and 6-1. Such changes deserve attention, especially if research is to continue its importance in medicine.

Table 6-15. Reactions of Medical Students in a National Representative Sample of Medical Schools in 1975 at Graduation and Matriculation

	Graduation June 1975 Class of 1975		Matriculation September 1975 Class of 1979	
	N	%	N	%
Reaction toward children:				
Negative	49	= 10.4	59	= 4.8
Neutral	98	= 20.8	187	= 15.3
Positive	323	= 68.7	982	= 80.0
Reaction toward young people:				
Negative	1	= 0.2	8	= 0.7
Neutral	49	= 10.5	170	= 13.9
Positive	419	= 89.3	1049	= 85.5
Reaction toward old people:				
Negative	63	= 14.5	122	= 10.0
Neutral	197	= 42.1	553	= 45.1
Positive	208	= 44.4	551	= 45.0

OTHER PROFESSIONALS AND
ALLIED HEALTH PERSONNEL

Professional health workers, such as nurses, nurse practitioners, psychologists, social workers, and allied health personnel, are changing their roles within medicine and consequently are demanding a significant voice in medical decisions as they affect the individual patient and medical care delivery. Most medical students would give other personnel a voice, but would reserve the final say to physicians. Resolution of the role of the physician in relation to these other workers is a primary issue for medicine. And in some groups, lawyers, educators, and welfare officials may also play a role.

GOVERNMENT SERVICE

These data show that few students would voluntarily work in a government service. Without a doctor draft, securing physicians for the armed services, prisons, indian reservations, Veterans Administration hospitals, and similar institutions has become almost impossible. Efforts such as a new U.S. Government Medical School, financial incentives in the form of a medical education, and loan programs with cancellation of debts in return for government service are promising programs that are being tried. This is a primary issue, especially when trying to accomplish this without reinstating the doctor draft. But working for the government clashes directly with students' desire to "be their own boss."

THE CONSUMER AND THE COMMUNITY
IN THE DELIVERY OF MEDICAL CARE

In general medicine, the roles of the consumer and of the community in deciding how medical care should be delivered are of major importance. What is unresolved is how this can best be accomplished. The majority of medical students would give the community and physicians an equal voice. This view is in marked contrast to that of older practitioners (see Table 6-16).

THE PHYSICIAN AS AN AGENT FOR
ATTACKING SOCIAL FACTORS

The data show that in recent years, a sizable number of medical students believe that the physician should be used to directly attack the social factors that are related to disease, and a small number

Table 6-16. Attitudes of Medical Students in a National Representative Sample of Medical Schools in 1975 at Graduation and Matriculation

Question: In the running of a neighborhood clinic, which of the following administrative arrangements do you prefer?	Graduation June 1975 Class of 1975		Matriculation September 1975 Class of 1979	
	N	%	N	%
Policy is decided by: Representatives of the community: physicians carry them out	21 =	4.4	34 =	2.8
The community and the physicians on an equal basis	276 =	58.0	715 =	58.5
The physicians, after consultation with the community	179 =	37.6	473 =	38.7

Table 6-17. Attitudes of Medical Students in a National Representative Sample of Medical Schools in 1975 at Graduation and Matriculation

Question: What things do you think you will like best about being a doctor?	Graduation June 1975 Class of 1975		Matriculation September 1975 Class of 1979	
	N	%	N	%
Being own boss: Very great or great	356 =	75.0	939 =	76.1
Some	95 =	20.0	240 =	19.5
Little or very little	24 =	5.1	55 =	4.5
Being able to change society Very great or great	106 =	22.5	396 =	32.1
Some	159 =	33.6	439 =	35.6
Little or very little	208 =	44.0	397 =	32.2

believe that medicine should be used to change society (see Table 6-17). The first group would use children with lead poisoning as the prototype. The physicians' principal function would be to work to get the paint off the walls through political action. This is not a new idea. In the 1890s, Sir William Osler attended every meeting of the Baltimore City Council for eight years to lobby for cleaning up the water system to decrease the cases of typhoid. He finally succeeded.

The second view is that the physician should actually use medicine to change society. Waitzkin and Modell[7] have discussed this point well. Table 6–14 shows that less than a majority of students, but more than would be expected, would be in favor of action prior to careful analysis of the problems.

SUMMARY

The attitudes of medical students at matriculation and graduation in 1975 in the national sample were discussed on a variety of pressing national issues, many of which are the subject of legislation.

The Manpower Act of 1976 which seeks to force medical students into careers in primary care and into medically underserviced geographic areas is having an effect. However, prior to the passage of this act, due to the law of supply and demand, students were moving in this direction. There is a question as to whether this act was necessary. In this movement, as for all students, the predominant mode of practice is group practice. The characteristics of students planning to practice in deprived areas were discussed.

Students are overwhelmingly in favor of other government legislation to insure the competence of physicians. Reference is made to the PSRO and laws requiring examinations or continuing medical education for relicensure.

On a number of miscellaneous issues of concern to the medical profession and society, medical students' attitudes were negative toward the "worried well" or patients with psychological problems and toward the aged and those in need of rehabilitation. Although most students saw the dehumanization of medicine as a problem of top priority, their attitudes would have to change for them to be instruments of a change to humanize medicine.

Few students would elect to work for the government; most would give an increasing voice to allied health workers and the consumer in deciding medical policies, reserving the final say to the physician. A small percentage see the physician's role as a social activist to change social factors that affect health and the delivery of medical care.

The attitudes of students toward research is not encouraging for the future of this enterprise. Only 2 percent would give it top priority as compared with 49 percent in the mid-sixties. Most students who would like a component of research in their careers are dubious of this possibility because of their perception that the funds will not be available.

Chapter 7

The Role of Medical Schools

The issue of what role the medical school should take in the changes affecting medical practice and the demands of society is far from resolved, especially for family physicians. An integral part of this dilemma concerns admissions and the medical school curriculum.

Since for the foreseeable future, the majority of graduates will have careers with a large component of primary care, the issue in admissions has shifted from: Can pressure be brought to bear on medical schools to select students who will follow such careers? to, Will the type of students that schools select be those who will function best in the new role? Will students be as humanistically oriented as needed to halt the depersonalization of care, or are there other students, who are presently denied admission, who would function better as family physicians?

Almost all medical schools are currently admitting more bioscientific than biosocial students (see Table 7-1). As mentioned, a sizable number of matriculating students had planned to go to graduate school in the sciences but changed careers during college because they no longer saw careers in science as viable. Fewer and fewer biosocial students, who are more humanistically oriented, gain admission.

The top priority for research in careers today is to determine whether students whose basic characteristics, career plans, and education are appropriate for one type of career will function as well in another career as those whose basic characteristics, plans, and education are more suitable to the career. Closely related to this

Table 7-1. The Orientations of Medical Students in a National Representative Sample of Medical Schools in 1975 at Graduation and Matriculation

	Graduation *June 1975* *Class of 1975*		*Matriculation* *September 1975* *Class of 1979*	
	N	*%*	*N*	*%*
Bioscientific	367 =	77.9	859 =	71.1
Biosocial	104 =	22.1	350 =	29.0

problem are two other important issues for admissions committees. The first is the importance of selecting students who will be flexible enough to change careers. The second issue is that with the probability of national health insurance, many observers are predicting that medicine will become more efficient and that the dehumanization of the patient and the physician will accelerate. Rogers[1] and Richardson[2] are both concerned about securing more humanistic care for patients. Rogers emphasizes selection and education to produce more humanistic care for patients, and Richardson emphasizes the institutional arrangements. Who is the culprit—the type of student admitted? the medical school itself? residencies? the practice of medicine? society itself? or a combination of all these factors?

Before research can supply any answers to the multiple problems of admissions, decisions will have to be made. Certainly, medical school faculty have decided to admit the scientists. But a negative correlation can be shown between humanistically oriented interests and scientists. There is often confusion over this, because the scientist is as interested in helping people as the biosocial student but plans to do so through science. The scientist cites that the poliomyelitis vaccine is far more "humanistic" than all the physicians who previously sat at the bedside of poliomyelitis patients. This, of course, is not an either/or problem; we need both types of physicians. There are emotional aspects of patients' illnesses that are important in medical care, and physicians must be prepared to handle them also if the patient is to improve. This is not meant to suggest the admission of only biosocial students. The great need for subspecialists and those to conduct research calls for the admission of sizable numbers of bioscientific students as well. Rather, it is a problem of proper balance.

Currently, the primary care group contains a mix of bioscientific and biosocial students rather than a preponderance of biosocial students, as was the case in the early seventies. If current admission policies continue, with the increasing admittance of bioscientific students, the relationship between basic characteristics of matriculating students and their careers at graduation can be projected to show even less relationship than is currently shown in Figure 2-5. The debate on this issue should proceed and, hopefully, some schools will experiment by admitting more biosocial students.

THE CURRICULUM AND INSTRUCTION IN MEDICAL SCHOOL

A fundamental problem regarding curriculum is whether the current practice of educating all medical students in the same way, except for some electives, is adequately preparing students for the type of career they will eventually have. Or, is such an education inappropriate for the large numbers of students who will be family practitioners? Should there be two curricula in medical schools, one for bioscientific students, leading to careers in academic medicine and subspecialties, and another for biosocial students who plan careers in family medicine, public health, or psychiatry? A committee of students at Harvard Medical School has worked out and proposed such a curriculum.[3] Student attitudes concerning this proposal are shown in Table 6-4.

Would a biosocial curriculum that would still be rigorous scientifically but with greater emphasis on psychiatry, public health, and the social and behavioral sciences educate physicians who would function better in primary care and psychiatry? Or is this a task for the residency or even beyond? Would such a curriculum result in physicians not competent enough in the technological aspects of medicine? Would a bioscientific curriculum, even more scientifically rigorous than current curricula, educate physicians who would function better as academicians and subspecialists? Or would such a curriculum result in doctors who are even less people- and humanistically oriented? Because of the economic pressures that will force many bioscientific students to have a large component of primary care in their practices, would the latter even be desirable? This is a tradeoff with no easy answers. Certainly, if many biosocial students are admitted, and the academic scientific demands continue to escalate as they normally do in response to the increasing ability and preparation in science of students in the courses, many of the biosocial students will have difficulty doing the work. One way to circumvent this is to select biosocial students who have more science background. In most cases, if they follow more advanced courses, their grades will be lower but they will be better prepared in science.

Unfortunately, there are data available that show that when medical schools place heavy emphasis on GPAs, the students who are admitted are actually less well prepared in the sciences because they take fewer science courses and lower level courses in order to insure a higher GPA.[4] If a firm policy were established whereby students better prepared in sciences (having taken more advanced courses) would be given preference in admissions over students with fewer courses and higher GPA's then obviously the preparation of biosocial students would increase, enabling them to do the work in a bioscientific curriculum.

Chapter 8

Conclusions

This study of medical students and physicians covered nineteen prospective years from 1958 to 1976, and nine retrospective years from 1949 to 1957, for a total of twenty-eight years. Data were collected at matriculation and graduation on Harvard medical students, and in some years, at the end of their second year; on these same students as alumni-alumnae in 1974-1975; on University of Michigan medical students from the class of 1973; and on a National Sample of Medical Students at graduation and matriculation in 1975.

One of the chief goals of the study was to determine if it is possible to predict from admission and matriculation data the career choices of students at graduation. The basic characteristics of students were determined by a number of techniques and each student was classified and then placed along a continuum that ranged from the predominantly bioscientific type to the predominantly biosocial type. Careers were also placed along a parallel continuum on the basis of the knowledge and skills that physicians use in a given career. Bioscientific careers included full- and part-time academic medicine and full-time specialty practice, especially subspecialty practice, excluding psychiatry. Biosocial careers included family medicine, public health, and psychiatry.

The societal factors affecting students were related to different eras of medicine: The Specialty Era of the fifties; the Scientific Era of the sixties; the Student Activism Era, 1969-1970; the Doldrums Era of the early seventies; and the current Primary Care and Increasing Governmental Control Era that began in 1975.

During the stable part of an era, it was possible to predict the career choices of students from admission and matriculation data at a highly statistically significant level. During unstable, transitional periods between eras and in the short-lived Student Activism Era, this was not possible. For example, during the Specialty, Scientific, and Doldrums Eras, it was possible to predict that bioscientific students at matriculation would follow bioscientific careers at graduation, and that biosocial students at entrance would follow biosocial careers at graduation. During the transition from the Specialty to the Scientific Era, this prediction was not possible. Although most bioscientific students followed bioscientific careers, many biosocial students took up bioscientific careers. During the brief Student Activism Era, many bioscientific students, because of the ideology of the times, elected biosocial careers, principally in community medicine and public health. But these career plans were as short-lived as the era itself, and the students reverted to bioscientific careers within two years. In the current new era, which represents a transition from the Doldrums Era to the Primary Care and Increasing Governmental Control Era, many bioscientific students are electing biosocial careers. Biosocial students still follow biosocial careers.

In short, when an era is stable and students perceive the economic viability of a career, and when ideology supports such a career, they follow their basic characteristics. However, when opportunities in careers are limited due to perceived or actual difficulties in funding or to ideological changes, then most students opt for the new careers regardless of their basic characteristics.

Economic incentives and ideology are more compelling for most students than their basic characteristics or original career plans. But both economic incentives and ideology must be present to insure career persistence. During the short-lived Student Activism Era, the ideology was present but the economic incentives were not, and the era quickly died. Currently, both the ideology and the funding are absent for careers in academic medicine and surgery, and less students elect such careers. Both the funding and ideology now support careers in primary care, and students respond, even if such careers do not conform to their basic characteristics.

The same predominant effects of societal factors are seen within the bioscientific and biosocial groups. For example, during the Specialty Era, most bioscientific students preferred full-time academic careers but correctly perceived that the funding would not support such careers and therefore planned part-time academic careers. During the Scientific Era, this same type of student could plan with confidence a full-time academic career because the ideology and funding supported such careers. Bioscientific students who had graduated late in the Specialty Era and were in residencies when the Scientific Era began quickly switched from part-time academic medicine to full-time academic medicine as such careers became more viable. In contrast, during the Scientific Era, biosocial students could no longer plan to become general or family practitioners as they could in the previous era because such a career was no longer viable. They opted for psychiatry because funding was available and the specialty was highly acceptable to society. The government supported this change in careers by offering economic incentives to established general practitioners to leave their practices and enter psychiatry residencies since it was felt that primary care practitioners were no longer needed. These places in psychiatry were oversubscribed by general practitioners.

During the Student Activism Era, there was a dramatic change in the career choices of biosocial students. From 100 percent of this group electing psychiatry at graduation, the majority changed to family medicine or public health, which suited their ideology. Students saw public health as a vehicle for social action leading to social change. The era quickly ended because of the lack of funding and because society, government, organized medicine, and medical schools refused to support it. Public health feel into disrepute by students because of their misconception that it was an opportunity to change society by attacking social factors related to health and disease. Currently, the large movement into family medicine and primary care is related to governmental action, economic viability, the ideology of the times, diminished funding for academic medicine, and the excessive numbers of surgeons and some subspecialists.

THE EFFECT OF THE MEDICAL SCHOOL ON CAREER CHOICES

The data collected in this study do not support the commonly held belief that a medical school is important in the career choices of its students. One of the most cherished ideas of the faculty has been their influence as role models on the career choices of their students. No data were found to support this. In none of the years of studying Harvard medical students, alumni-alumnae, or the National Sample of Students did more than 18 percent of the students feel that anyone on the faculty had influenced their choice of career (see Table 8-1).

Then too, the movement of students into various careers, except

Table 8-1.   Specialty Choice of Medical Students in a National Representative Sample of Medical Schools in 1975 at Graduation and Matriculation

	Graduation June 1975 Class of 1975		Matriculation September 1975 Class of 1979	
	N	%	N	%
Psychiatry	19 =	4.0	26 =	2.2
Other	452 =	96.0	1183 =	97.8
Totals	471* =	100	1209** =	100

*Eight respondents out of 479 did not indicate a specialty choice at graduation.
**Thirty-five respondents out of 1,242 did not indicate a specialty choice at matriculation.

during the Scientific Era, was at variance with the wishes of the faculty. During that era, society, government, and students all embraced science, which had the highest national priority. Ideology and funding supported these career choices, but the faculty took great credit for it. However, when students changed careers during the Student Activism Era, the Doldrums Era, and the current era, their choices were different from those of the faculty and again more related to ideology and funding. This was best seen in surgery, where for many years the faculty boasted of their influence on the many students choosing surgery. Recently, with surgery being such a difficult career to follow due to the excessive numbers of practitioners, the number of students electing surgery has decreased markedly. But the faculty and the teaching have remained the same.

Other data relate to the effect of curriculum changes on career choices. One of the chief reasons for changing the curriculum was to alter the career choices of students. There was no change in the curriculum at the Harvard Medical School in 1958 when the marked change toward careers in academic medicine began, with students placing their highest priority on research. Had the curriculum been changed at that time, many would have attributed the changes to the curriculum change.

The curriculum was changed in 1968 to give students more opportunities in science. It was also in that year that the marked change away from academic medicine toward family medicine began. This change was contrary to the wishes of the faculty. The experience at Duke was similar.[1]

At the present time, government is trying to redistribute the career choices and geographic practice location of physicians by increasing regulation of medical schools. It is clear from the data gathered on this project that this is doomed to failure. Factors outside of the medical school, such as economic incentives and ideology, are the leading factors in the career choices of medical students. The only exception is that admittance of a higher percentage of students who are reared in rural areas will result in a higher number of physicians in rural areas, but here it is only 50 percent. The task of the medical school is to have the freedom to educate physicians to their highest degree of skill. It is the task of government to make this possible. Competence in medicine will be assured this way. Redistribution of physicians in specialties must come from outside of the medical schools in economic incentives and the law of supply and demand. The data on this project support the above statements.

LIFESTYLE, VALUES, AND VARIABLES IN CAREER CHOICE

Throughout the years, lifestyle has affected women far more than men in choice of career. However, data collected at matriculation on the national sample suggest that this is no longer a factor for women. They now choose the same careers as men.

The significant change in lifestyle is that nearly all students wish to work fewer hours and to have more time for their families and for outside activities. This they see as best accomplished by group practice, and over 95 percent of the students currently plan this type of practice. Only secondarily do they see group practice as a means for improving the quality or lowering the cost of medical care.

Decline in the number of hours students plan to work will be an important factor in determining the number of physicians needed for the future. Clearly, if most physicians work far fewer hours, more will be needed unless the practice of medicine becomes more efficiently organized and more involved with physician extenders and technological aids such as computers. In addition, over 80 percent of students in the national sample see the "dehumanization" of patients as a major problem, particularly if physicians work even fewer hours, contributing to a further loss of personal attention to patients.

An important variable studied in career choice was that of values.

During each of the eras, values changed concomitant with the chief social responsibility of physicians (see Table 2-1). During the Specialty Era, most students emphasized competence; during the Scientific Era, research; during the Student Activism Era, the delivery of medical care; during the Doldrums Era, again competence, which in the current era is also placed first by students.

The change in some of these values is striking; the decline in the percentage placing research in first place with a rating of 49 percent during the Scientific Era to the current rating of 2 percent is ominous for the future of science. The change toward emphasizing the importance of the delivery of medical care, especially by those electing careers in primary care, and the emphasis on preventive medicine by students planning to practice in deprived areas, are strong current trends. These values are consonant with the eras in which they developed.

All of the variables examined for their effects on career choices showed significant influence except for the effect of the medical school experience itself. The predominant variable was that of societal factors outside of the medical school, which include economic incentives and ideology. The predominance of societal factors on career choices of students can best be seen by studying the changes in career choices of medical students in the same year, whether they were in the first, second, or senior year (see Figure 3-1). This shows that changes occurred in the same direction, in the same year, simultaneously in freshmen, sophomores, and seniors.

Further evidence of the striking effect of societal factors were studies of the pool of applicants to the Harvard Medical School over two four year periods, 1959-1963 and 1968-1972. The pool contained students from all states and from more than 240 different colleges. Examination of their transcripts showed that in 1959, after the launching of Sputnik, freshmen, sophomores, juniors, and seniors began simultaneously to study more science, whether they were in New England, the South, the Far West, or the Middle West. In 1968, examination of students' transcripts showed that applicants everywhere and in all four years of college began to study the social sciences. The percentage in the pool taking a social science course rose from 20 percent to 78 percent in one year and then to over 90 percent.

These changes occurred in the same years that students in all four classes in medical school changed their career choices—in 1959 to more bioscientific careers; in 1969 to more biosocial careers. These simultaneous, parallel changes in all four classes in medical school and in four college classes throughout the country cannot be explained in any other way except that they were the result of societal factors outside of medical schools and colleges.

PRIMARY CARE: A SUMMARY

Extensive studies were made on the characteristics of students who elected careers in primary care. The term primary care is a recent one, so that different criteria were used in different eras. During the Specialty Era, it was general practice; during the Scientific Era, too few students elected such careers to make studies of seniors, but it was possible to study those students who chose general practice at matriculation which they abandoned during medical school. During the Student Activism Era, primary care was considered family or community medicine; during the Doldrums Era, it was family medicine; and currently, primary care is considered to be general internal medicine, general pediatrics, and family medicine.

Just as in career choices in general, the characteristics of purveyors of primary care were easy to delineate in stable eras, and difficult in the transitions between eras. During the Specialty Era, they had the characteristics of the student-practitioner. Their chief interest was in working directly with people, using science pragmatically to solve medical problems. Compared with other medical students, they had lower grades, markedly lower MCAT scores, and less science preparation. During the Scientific Era, students who entered planning to become general practitioners had the same characteristics as students in this group in the previous era, but by graduation, almost all opted for psychiatry. During the Doldrums Era, the students in primary care, as contrasted with students who elected other careers, had biosocial characteristics. They had measured interests in interpersonal relationships and human behavior rather than science. They had lower quantitative and science scores on the MCAT; were nonscience majors; were less interested in status, prestige, and financial rewards; and scored lower than bioscientific students on all parts of the national boards except psychiatry.

In contrast to the highly significant relationship of the basic characteristics at matriculation to career choices at graduation during the stable eras, few significant relationships were found during the transitional eras or during the brief, unstable Student Activism Era. During the transition from the Specialty to the Scientific Era, many biosocial students changed their characteristics to those of bioscientific students, and many who did not make these changes abandoned general practice for psychiatry. During the

Student Activism Era, many bioscientific students elected careers in family medicine or public health, which they quickly gave up when academic careers were seen as more viable two years later. During the current transition into the Primary Care and Increasing Governmental Control Era, many bioscientific students are choosing careers in primary care, thus joining their biosocial colleagues, making for a mixture that turns highly significant differences in characteristics into trends. Whether these bioscientific students will revert to their original bioscientific career choices, which they still prefer, will depend upon whether or not those career choices become economically feasible. What will happen to their performance as physicians if they are blocked by economic factors from becoming surgeons, cardiologists, and certain other specialists and subspecialists where there are excessive numbers of practitioners remains to be seen. Will they perform at a high level if they are forced to stay in careers they do not prefer and careers that do not correspond to their basic characteristics?

The data collected during the transition from the Specialty Era to the Scientific Era are relevant here. At that time, many biosocial students elected bioscientific careers. Many changed their characteristics to those of bioscientific students, others compromised by entering psychiatry, and still others elected new careers that did not correspond to their basic characteristics and became embittered. Based on those data, bioscientific students currently forced into primary care will either change their characteristics to those of biosocial students and be content in their new careers, will compromise, or will become embittered. The compromise is to practice general internal medicine with special attention to a subspecialty, with the hope that conditions will change so that the physician can devote himself full-time to his subspecialty.

The general public, in a nostalgic way, would like medical schools to select students in the model of the general practitioners of bygone eras. The data on this project show that when students electing general practice in the fifties were compared with students in the physician associate program at Duke in 1973, they were found to be remarkably similar. Given the advance in the scientific aspects of medicine and the increasing attention to the social aspects of medicine, today's biosocial student is far more suited to the practice of the future than the general practitioner of the fifties.

DEPRIVED AREAS

Until recently, it was difficult to study the characteristics of students planning to practice in medically deprived areas because so few did.

During the Specialty and Scientific Eras, they were nearly all women. Almost all planned to or practiced in slums. Currently, both at Harvard and in the national sample in 1975, there are sufficient students—25 percent to 30 percent—who plan to practice in deprived areas to make analyses. Almost all are in family practice and plan to practice in rural areas, few in slums (see Tables 6-4, 6-5, and 6-6). These students differ from those interested in primary care but not planning to practice in deprived areas, in that they are predominantly family practitioners rather than pediatricians or internists, were born and reared in rural areas, place greater emphasis on preventive medicine and public health in their practice, and plan to be more politically active on medical care delivery problems. They are similar to other primary care physicians not planning to practice in deprived areas in certain characteristics, but these characteristics are more marked in this group. Reference is made to their interest in interpersonal relationships and behavioral problems rather than science; their lower quantitative and science MCAT scores; their lower national board scores on all subjects in both Part I and Pat II, with the exception of psychiatry; and their lack of emphasis on status, prestige, and financial rewards. There was no sex difference between primary care physicians planning to practice in deprived areas and those who do not plan such practices. In the alumni/alumnae sample, significantly more men were in rural areas and more women in slums. Medical students in 1975 planning to practice in deprived areas show no difference. Most plan rural areas; very few slums.

WOMEN

The data on women showed marked changes in career choices and attitudes over the years. In the fifties and sixties, almost all of the women admitted to medical school had biosocial characteristics, and most often they chose careers in pediatrics, psychiatry, or general internal medicine. Although never high, a greater percentage of women than men worked in slums.

Beginning in the early seventies, with the onset of the feminist movement, the career choices of women changed until, in the national matriculation sample in 1975, there were no significant differences in career choices between women and men. There were slightly more women in obstetrics-gynecology, but this was only a trend. This resulted from some decrease in women choosing biosocial careers but a concomitant increase in men choosing biosocial careers. More striking, and indicating a fundamental change, was that there was no significant difference in the percentage of women and men choosing pediatrics, where in the past this had been the greatest difference between the careers of the sexes.

The most significant change in women's attitudes was that formerly a very high percentage felt that there were marked prejudices against them by male physicians; currently few women medical students feel that such prejudices exist. Surprisingly, throughout the years, only a small percentage of women felt that having a family had impeded their careers; indeed, certain women felt that marriage had increased their options because, in making career choices, they did not have to consider finances because of their husbands' income. The same percentage of men as women felt that having a family had interfered with their careers since they had been forced to make career decisions, not in their best interests, but based on financial considerations.

Currently, women come from families of equal social status to those of male medical students, not superior as in the past, and no longer do their mothers have more education and careers. They make equal grades in the sciences, although they still plan to earn less money and to work fewer hours than men. If we consider the number of hours women expect to work as compared to men and project this twenty-five years beyond medical school, women are only two work years behind men. However, if we project this onto the longevity of women at that age, women will work longer, in numbers of years, than men. This is a rough projection, but it does suggest that the idea that women physicians work less than men is a myth.

The major question women and men debate with regard to the increasing number of women in medicine is whether women bring something special to medicine. Both men and women differ in their opinions. Some feel that women are no different than men professionally and should be considered as physicians only; others feel that women bring something special to medicine that men cannot.

MINORITY GROUP STUDENTS

Increasing numbers of minority group students are entering medical school, although the numbers are not yet as large as was originally planned. It is important that special efforts be expended to increase minority group programs because these students bring much to medicine. These data show increased preparation on the part of these students as larger numbers have gained access to better secondary school and college educations. In time, there will be no need for these special programs. But until then, the programs should be accelerated.

Residency and hospital appointments should be expanded for these minority students. Unfortunately the burden for the solution of the delivery of medical care to deprived areas is often placed on minority group students. This is a poor solution to the problem because they cannot solve it alone and because it might push them into careers for which they are not suited or prevent them from pursuing those for which they are best suited. Moreover, unless each is free to follow his or her interests and abilities, these programs will fail. Minority group students must eventually ascend to leadership positions and have power in the medical hierarchy; otherwise things will not change drastically.

Minority group students alone cannot now provide adequate medical care in deprived areas because of the long lead time—at least fifteen years—before a sufficient number of them will have graduated and received their training. This is an evasion of the problem that belongs to the majority, even more than to the minority, because it was the majority that created the problem.

While minority group students must be free to follow their own careers, in a practical vein, little will be accomplished unless those who concern themselves directly with the problems of the delivery of medical care to their people, and those who choose careers within medicine not directly related to the delivery of medical care, continue to press the medical profession for action. There is abundant evidence that, left to themselves, government, medical schools, and the profession will not act to acquire the necessary balance within medicine to see that the diverse needs of society are met. Since 1965, thousands of medical students have received federal loans which can be cancelled by serving two years in a medically deprived area; yet very few have done so.[2]

A QUESTION FOR TODAY

The critical question today, with the onset of the new Primary Care and Increasing Governmental Control Era, is not whether many medical students will have careers in primary care. It is already apparent that they will. The question is whether, in following a career that many of them did not choose and that does not correspond to their basic characteristics, they will be satisfied, effective practitioners of primary care, or be embittered and discontent and as a result practice poor medicine?

Another change in medicine that may affect the performance of physicians, regardless of specialty, is the effect of increasing governmental controls. The conditions under which a physician practices and the location of practice will come under increasing government regulation, a fact resented by most physicians. In the questionnaire used in the project, many checked that one of the things they liked about being a physician is "being my own boss." We can predict that some physicians will embrace the new conditions, others will compromise, and still others will become embittered.

Both of these conditions—practicing in a specialty the physician did not prefer and increasing governmental controls—may affect physician performance. The data collected on this project is in accord with the hypothesis of the German sociologist Max Weber, who postulated that

> A direct relationship exists between the form of an economic or social organization and the type of individual necessary to create and perpetuate it. When institutions change, those who functioned successfully in the old system often find themselves unable to cope with the new set of circumstances and are gradually succeeded by other individuals with different values, attitudes, and abilities, who are better equipped to function in the new system. For example, there is a widely observable phenomenon that as the need for new skills and abilities arises within a culture, men and women with the requisite skills appear to fill these roles. Thus, in our society, as science became more important, within ten years the number of scientists increased markedly, until today there are more living scientists than in all of past history.[3]

Although Weber's hypothesis has proven true in the United States in the past, it is impossible to predict how much disruption will occur in medicine as physicians are called upon to assume new careers they did not choose. Also, with the huge increase in the population of college and graduate students in recent years, there are large numbers of graduates who will be unable to find jobs commensurate with their educations, resulting in mass underemployment. It is estimated that as many as 70 percent to 80 percent of recent graduates will be underemployed. In many other countries, this has resulted in social upheaval. The changes in the ability of physicians to choose their careers freely is thus a reflection of what is taking place in society as a whole.

It is imperative that research into career determinants continue, with emphasis on the function of physicians in careers they did not choose. The task is to determine which factors in physicians and within medical schools and beyond facilitate and impede high performance in careers. On the basis of such data, an improved admission program and better counseling of medical students could be instituted. As we enter the new Primary Care and Increasing

Governmental Control Era, we can already see the harbingers of change in the medical students who will function in the new system.

It is apparent that as medicine changes from one era to the next, frequently the pendulum swings too far in the new direction, often wiping out the gains from the previous eras. For example, the shift from the Specialty to the Scientific Era beginning in 1959 built the academic medical center, one of the great accomplishments of medicine. But at the same time this shift resulted in the neglect of the delivery of primary care, particularly in deprived areas. Will the shift now into primary care and increasing governmental control again go so far that science will have to be rediscovered some ten or fifteen years hence? The low priority given research by today's medical students, down from 49 percent as a top priority in 1963 to 2 percent in 1976, is ominous. The crucial question is how to achieve a balance in what society needs from the medical profession. Otherwise, George Bernard Shaw's quotation is apt: "You think you are making progress because there is so much movement, when in truth you are merely swinging on a pendulum."[4]

Eras are becoming shorter and shorter in duration, making planning difficult. Before one set of plans can be implemented, the circumstances change. The basic premise of this study is that if effective planning is to take place for medicine in the future, as hazardous as predictions are in view of ever more rapid social changes, they can be more accurate if data are used and we accept Lincoln's statement: "If we know where we have been, where we are now, and the direction in which we are tending, we may make a better decision." Hopefully, this study, which gives a view of the past twenty-eight years of medicine as it affects the careers of medical students and physicians, can have some effect on that planning.

Notes

CHAPTER 1

1. D.K. Price, *The Scientific Estate* (Cambridge, Massachusetts: Harvard University Press, 1965).
2. D.H. Funkenstein, Medical Students, Medical Schools and Society During Three Eras of Medical Education, in R.H. Combs and C.E. Vincent, eds., *Psychosocial Aspects of Medical Training* (Springfield, Illinois: C.C. Thomas, 1971).
3. H. Brooks, Can Science Survive in the Modern Age? *Science* 174:21-30 (1970).
4. Carnegie Council On Policy Studies in Higher Education, *Progress and Problems in Medical and Dental Education: Federal Support Versus Federal Control*, A Report of the Carnegie Council on Policy Studies in High Education (San Francisco: Jossey-Bass, 1976).

CHAPTER 2

1. A.E. Severinghaus; H.J. Carman; and W.E. Jr. Cadbury, *Preparation for Medical Education in the Liberal Arts College* (New York: McGraw-Hill, 1953); and A.E. Severinghaus; H.J. Carman; and W.E., Jr. Cadbury, *Preparation for Medical Education: A Restudy* (New York: McGraw-Hill, 1961).
2. D.H. Funkenstein, Medical Students, Medical Schools and Society During Three Eras of Medical Education, in R.H. Combs and C.E. Vincent, eds., *Psychosocial Aspects of Medical Training* (Springfield, Illinois: C.C. Thomas, 1971).
3. P.J. Sanazaro, *Educational Self Study by Schools of Medicine* (Evanston, Illinois: Association of American Medical Colleges, 1967).
4. D.H. Funkenstein, A New Breed of Psychiatrist? *Am. J. of Psychiatry* 124:226-28 (1967).

5. W.F. Duke, and D.G. Johnson, Study of U.S. Medical School Applicants 1974-75, J. of Med. Educat 51:877-896, 1976.

6. M.J.K. McKusick; K.D. Anderson; and P.K. Garrison, What It's Been Like, *Harvard Med. Alumni Bull.* 48:20-23 (1974).

7. R.B. Freeman, *The Over-Educated American* (New York: Academic Press, 1976).

8. J.A.D. Cooper, 1977 Matching Announced: Activities at AAMC, Weekly Report No. 77-10 (Washington, D.C.: Association of American Medical Colleges, March 14, 1977).

9. D.H. Funkenstein, Medical Students, Medical Schools and Society During Three Eras of Medical Education, in R.H. Combs and C.E. Vincent, eds., *Psychosocial Aspects of Medical Training* (Springfield, Illinois: C.C. Thomas, 1971).

CHAPTER 3

1. H. Brooks, Can Science Survive in the Modern Age? *Science* 174:21-30 (1970).

CHAPTER 4

1. D.H. Funkenstein, The Implications of Diversity of Medical Students, in *The Ecology of the Medical Student*, ch. 2, a Report of the Fifth Teaching Institute (Evanston, Illinois: Association of American Medical Colleges, 1958).

2. C.F. Schumacher, Personal Characteristics of Students Choosing Different Types of Medical Careers, *J. of Med. Educat.* 39:278-88 (1964).

3. P.J. Sanazaro, *Educational Self Study by Schools of Medicine* (Evanston, Illinois: Association of American Medical Colleges, 1967).

4. F.J. Lyden; H.J. Geiger; and O.L. Peterson, *The Training of Good Physicians* (Cambridge, Massachusetts: Harvard University Press, 1968).

5. D.H. Funkenstein, A New Breed of Psychiatrist? *Am. J. of Psychiatry* 124:226-28 (1967).

6. D.H. Funkenstein, The Problem of Increasing the Number of Psychiatrists, *Am. J. of Psychiat.* 121:852 (1965).

7. Schumacher, pp. 278-88.

8. Bulletin of Duke University 1972-1973 Physicians Associate Program (Durham, North Carolina).

9. E. Crovitz; N.M. Huse; and D.E. Lewis, Selection of Physicians Assistants, *J. of Med. Educat.* 48:551-55 (1973).

10. I. Berg, *Education and Jobs: The Great Training Robbery* (Boston: Beacon Press, 1971).

11. C.A. Janeway, Family Medicine—Fad or Need? *New Eng. J. of Med.* 291:337-43 (1974).

12. E.S. Caveny, and E.A. Strecker, Subsequent Nation-wide Effects of World War II Navy Psychiatric Training Program, *Am. J. of Psychiat.* 109:481 (1953); and G.A. Forrer, and J. Grisell, U.S. Army Psychiatric Training Program: Subsequent Nation-wide Effects, *Arch. Neurol. & Psychiat.* 77:220 (1957).

13. E. Ginsberg, *Men, Money and Medicine* (New York: Columbia University Press, 1969).

14. D.H. Funkenstein, Medical Students, Medical Schools and Society During Three Eras of Medical Education, in R.H. Combs and C.E. Vincent, eds., *Psychosocial Aspects of Medical Training* (Springfield, Illinois: C.C. Thomas, 1971).

CHAPTER 5

1. The First Decade of Women in the Harvard Medical School, 1949-1959 (Boston: Harvard Medical Alumni Association, 1959).

2. D.H. Funkenstein; S.H. King; and M.E. Drolette, *Mastery of Stress* (Cambridge, Massachusetts: Harvard University Press, 1957).

3. M.J.K. McKusick; K.D. Anderson; and P.K. Garrison, What It's Been Like, *Harvard Med. Alumni Bull.* 48:20-23 (1974).

CHAPTER 6

1. J.A.D. Cooper, 1977 Matching Announced: Activities at AAMC, Weekly Report No. 77-10 (Washington, D.C.: Association of American Medical Colleges, March 14, 1977).

2. California Medical Association, Bureau of Research and Planning, Division of Socioeconomics and Research, A Survey of Attitudes of Medical Students and Recent Graduates (San Francisco, 1973).

3. S.R. Garfield, The Delivery of Medical Care, *Sci. Am.* 4:222, (1970).

4. E.L. Richardson, Shattuck Lecture, "The Old Order Changeth, Yielding Place to the New: Perspectices of the Health Revolution," *New Eng. J. of Med.* 291:283-87 (1974).

5. D.E. Rogers, Health Care and the Academic Center, *The Pharos of Alpha Omega Alpha* 36:49-54, (1973).

6. Richardson, pp. 283-87.

7. H. Waitzkin and H. Modell, Medicine, Socialism and Totalitarianism: Lessons from Chile, *New Eng. J. of Med.* 291:171-77, (1974).

CHAPTER 7

1. D.E. Rogers, Health Care and the Academic Center, *The Pharos of Alpha Omega Alpha* 36:49-54, (1973).

2. E.L. Richardson, Shattuck Lecture, "The Old Order Changeth, Yielding Place to the New: Perspectices of the Health Revolution," *New Eng. J. of Med.* 291:283-87 (1974).

CHAPTER 8

1. J.J. Preiss, Some Responses of Medical Students to Training Programs and to the Professions, *J. of Med. Educat.* 49:8 (1974).

2. D.H. Funkenstein, *Advising Minority Students Enrolled in Medical School* (New York: The Macy Foundation and National Medical Fellowships Inc., 1973).

3. M. Weber, *The Theory of Social and Economic Organization* (Part I of *Wirtschaft und Gessellschaft*), translated from the German by A.R. Henderson and T. Parsons (Cambridge, Massachusetts. Talcott Parsons, 1942).

4. G.B. Shaw, *Man and Superman* (New York: Longmans, Green and Company, 1956).

Appendixes

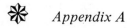 *Appendix A*

Matriculation Questionnaire For Entering Freshmen

MATRICULATION QUESTIONNAIRE
FOR ENTERING FRESHMEN.

_____(1-5,6)

NAME_____

MEDICAL SCHOOL_____

TODAY'S DATE_____

SEX: (Check one)   Male_____1
                                           Female_____2   (8)

AGE: (Indicate years)   _____ (9-10)

MARITAL STATUS: (Check one)   Single_____1
                                           Married_____2
                                           Divorced_____3   (11)
                                           Separated____4

CHILDREN: (Check one)   Yes_____1
                                           No_____2   (12)

129

1. What is your father's occupation? Be specific. (If retired or deceased, record this fact and indicate his former occupation.)

    _____ (17)

2. What is your father's education? (Circle highest level attained)

    GRADE SCHOOL   HIGH SCHOOL   COLLEGE   POST-GRADUATE
    1 2 3 4 5 6 7 8   9 10 11 12   13 14 15 16   17 18 19 20 and over   (18-19)

3. What is your mother's education? (Circle highest level attained)

    GRADE SCHOOL   HIGH SCHOOL   COLLEGE   POST-GRADUATE
    1 2 3 4 5 6 7 8   9 10 11 10   13 14 15 16   17 18 19 20 and over   (20-21)

4. What is your mother's present occupation? Be specific.

    If Housewife, check here_____1 _____ (22)

5. Which of the following best describes the place where you grew up?
    (Check one)

                                       A farm or ranch_____1
                            A town of less than 10,000_____2
             A small city of from 10,000 to 100,000_____3
                              A suburb of a large city_____4   (23)
                                    Within a large city_____5
        You moved so much it would be hard to say_____6

6. Is or was your mother or father a doctor?

                                            Neither_____1
                                             Mother_____2
                                             Father_____3   (24)
                                               Both_____4

7. Did you ever interrupt your undergraduate college education for a year or
    more? (Check one)

                                                Yes_____1
                                                 No_____2   (25)

8. Indicate how many summers you worked in the following areas before
    medical school:

                          Hospital work with patients_____
             Lab assistant or technician in a hospital_____
                                           Research_____   (26-30)
                     Work in slums or rural areas_____
                                              Other_____
        What?_____

9. How many summers was it necessary for you to earn money to support yourself as an undergraduate in college?

                                          none _____ 0
                                             1 _____ 1
                                             2 _____ 2
                                             3 _____ 3   (31)
                                             4 _____ 4

10. Did you have to work to support yourself during the academic year as an undergraduate at college (excluding summers)?

                                           Yes _____ 1
                                            No _____ 2   (33)

11. From which type of secondary school were you graduated? (Check one)

                                        Public _____ 1
                                       Private _____ 2   (35)
                                     Parochial _____ 3

12. <u>Rank</u> the following subjects according to the amount of pleasure they gave you during college by writing "1" for the most enjoyable subject, <u>and so on</u> to "4" for the least enjoyable subject.

                              Rank assigned

              Natural sciences _____
           Behavioral sciences _____
                    Humanities _____   (36-39)
               Social sciences _____

13. Did you do any research while an undergraduate at college?

                                           Yes _____ 1
                                            No _____ 2   (40)

14. If you did any research during college, specify which field: (Check the
predominant field)

$$
\begin{array}{lr}
\text{Biology} & 1 \\
\text{Chemistry} & 2 \\
\text{Biochemistry} & 3 \\
\text{Engineering or Physical Science} & 4 \\
\text{Public Health} & 5 \\
\text{Social Sciences} & 6 \\
\text{Behavioral Sciences} & 7 \\
\text{Other} & 8 \\
\text{What?} & \\
\end{array}
$$

(42)

15. If you had not been going to medical school, would you have preferred
to major in something else while in college? (Check one)

$$
\begin{array}{lr}
\text{Yes} & 1 \\
\text{No} & 2 \\
\end{array}
$$

(44)

If the answer is yes, would it have been:
(Check one)

$$
\begin{array}{lr}
\text{A Science} & 1 \\
\text{Humanities} & 2 \\
\text{Social Science} & 3 \\
\text{Psychology} & 4 \\
\text{Don't Know} & 5 \\
\text{Other - What?} & 6 \\
\end{array}
$$

(45)

If the answer is yes, did you elect your
college major because: (Check one)

A   The curriculum in my college was so set
up that this major allowed me to take
the electives that I wanted   1

B. I thought it the best way to get into
medical school   2   (46)

C. I thought it the best way to prepare
for medical school   3

D. I made an understandable mistake   4

E. It was the subject I was most
interested in   5

16. Before deciding on medicine, did you ever seriously consider any other occupation or profession? (Check one)

$$\text{Yes} \underline{\qquad} 1$$
$$\text{No} \underline{\qquad} 2 \qquad (47)$$

If _yes_, did you ever consider a career in one or more of the following fields? (Check as many as apply)

Sciences, PhD level_____

Humanities, PhD level_____

Social Sciences, PhD level_____

Psychology, PhD level_____

Becoming a businessman or woman_____

Becoming a lawyer_____

Becoming a teacher of elementary
or secondary school_____   (48-60)

Becoming a Social Worker_____

Going to a School of Public Health_____

Becoming a Hospital Administrator_____

Becoming a dentist_____

Becoming an engineer or
architect_____

Other, What?_____

17. Did you have difficulty in making up your mind whether to pursue an M.D. or PhD?

$$\text{Yes} \underline{\qquad} 1 \qquad (61)$$
$$\text{No} \underline{\qquad} 2$$

If _yes_, which of the following areas did you consider for a PhD? (Check one)

Natural Sciences_____ 1

Behavioral Sciences_____ 2   (62)

Humanities_____ 3

Social Sciences_____ 4

18. If on **several attempts**, you had **failed** to secure entrance to any **medical** school would you have: (Check one)

> Gone to graduate schools in the natural
> sciences_____1
> Gone to graduate school in the humanities_____2
> Gone to graduate school in the social
> sciences_____3
> Gone to graduate school in psychology_____4
> Become a businessman_____5
> Become a Lawyer_____6
> Become a teacher of elementary or
> secondary school_____7   (63-64)
> Gone to Dental School_____8
> Gone to Social Work School_____9
> Gone to a School of Public Health_____10
> Become a Hospital Administrator_____11
> Become an Engineer or Architect_____12
> Other, What?_____13

19. When did you <u>first</u> think of becoming a physician? (Check one)

> Before college_____1
> First two years of college_____2
> Junior year_____3   (65)
> Senior year_____4
> After college_____5

20. When did you <u>consolidate</u> your career plans to become a physician? (Check one)

> Before college_____1
> First two years of college_____2
> Junior year_____3   (66)
> Senior year_____4
> After college_____5

21. <u>Rank</u> the following subjects according to the grades you received in them in college by writing "1" for the highest grades, "2" for the next, and so on to "4".

> Rank assigned
>
> Natural sciences_____
> Behavioral sciences_____   (67-70)
> Humanities_____
> Social sciences_____

22. What was your college major or field of concentration? (Check one)

Biochemical Sciences _____ 1
Biochemistry _____ 2
Biology _____ 3
Biophysics _____ 4
Chemistry _____ 5
Cultural Anthropology _____ 6
Economics _____ 7   (71-72)
Engineering _____ 8
Government or Political Science _____ 9
Humanities _____ 10
Mathematics _____ 11
Physics _____ 12
Pre-Med _____ 13
Psychology _____ 14
Sociology _____ 15

23. When you entered college did you plan to: (Check one)

Become a physician _____ 1
Go to graduate school in the sciences _____ 2
Go to graduate school in the humanities _____ 3
Go to graduate school in the social
sciences _____ 4
Go to graduate school in psychology _____ 5
Become a businessman _____ 6
Become a lawyer _____ 7
Become a teacher of elementary or _____   (73-74)
secondary school _____ 8
Go to dental school _____ 9
Go to social work school _____ 10
Go to a school of public health _____ 11
Become a hospital administrator _____ 12
Become an engineer or architect _____ 13
Undecided _____ 14
Other, What? _____ 15

Col. 80-1

The following vignettes are descriptions of various careers of physicians. Please read them carefully since you will be asked to answer questions about the one which best corresponds to your future career.

CAREER NUMBER 1

This physician is in one of the clinical specialities such as medicine, surgery, pediatrics, neurology, etc. He or she is highly specialized in one of the subspecialties of a major specialty. For example, if an internist, he or she is a gastroenterologist, a kidney specialist, a pulmonary specialist, an endocrinologist, etc. If a surgeon, he or she is an orthopedic surgeon, a plastic surgeon, an abdominal surgeon, a thoracic surgeon, etc.

This physician is an excellent scientist and his or her education is basically biological. This doctor is affiliated with a medical school on a part-time basis, doing some teaching, but his or her major activity is the practice of medicine. This doctor is so busy with his or her patient load that although he or she would like to, he or she can spend little time on the emotional, social, and family aspects of the patients's illnesses. A clinical professor describes this physician.

CAREER NUMBER 2

This doctor is in one of the subspecialties of a major specialty, similar to the physician in Career 1. However, this physician is full-time with a medical school in which he or she devotes about 70% of his or her time to research, often in a basic science. He or she has minor teaching duties and spends approximately 30% of his or her time in patient care, hospital based, which is largely carried out by supervising residents. "Academic medicine" is applied to this type of career.

CAREER NUMBER 3

This physician is full-time with a medical school. After graduation from medical school, he or she was a post-doctoral fellow for two years in one of the basic medical sciences and now teaches and does research full-time in a medical school in a basic medical science. He or she has no clinical practice.

CAREER NUMBER 4

This doctor is in one of the clinical specialties and may or may not be in a subspecialty. He or she is not affiliated with a medical school but with an excellent community hospital. This doctor has a full-time private practice.

CAREER NUMBER 5

This physician majored in college in a physical science such as mathematics, computers, engineering, or physics, and has a career involving various mixtures of research, teaching and patient care. This doctor is mainly concerned with medical problems which involve his or her knowledge of these sciences. These would include applying computers to medicine, systems analysis, biomedical engineering, artificial organs, cardiac monitoring, etc.

CAREER NUMBER 6

This doctor is a psychiatrist. He or she is either full-time with a medical school or affiliated with one, works in a community clinic or in a full-time private practice. This physician is primarily concerned with research and/or treatment of patients with psychiatric problems.

CAREER NUMBER 7

This physician is a Public Health Physician. He or she is primarily concerned with the prevention of bacteriological diseases and works in a governmental agency.

CAREER NUMBER 8

This doctor is a new type of Public Health Physician with his or her major basis in the social sciences, particularly economics, ecology, and ethnology. He or she is either doing research in improving the methods for the delivery of medical care and/or administering such a system, either hospital or community based.

CAREER NUMBER 9

This physician is a new type of Public Health Physician with a basis in behavioral sciences, such as social psychology, sociology, and cultural anthropology. He or she deals with the problems of diseases which are "man-made and environmental" such as auto accidents, air and water pollution, alcoholism, drug addiction, smoking, etc. This doctor deals with human behavior on a community wide basis. He or she may do research alone, administer programs in this area, or a combination of research and administration.

CAREER NUMBER 10

This doctor is engaged in the family practice of medicine. His or her training is in one of two specialties, internal medicine or pediatrics. In addition to training in his or her basic specialty, this physician has some training in psychiatry and public health. This doctor treats all members of the family, not only paying attention to their physical problems, but also to the emotional, social, and family aspects of their illnesses. Extremely complicated or unusual problems are referred to physicians in subspecialties.

CAREER NUMBER 11

This physician is the new Primary Physician with training in internal medicine, pediatrics, psychiatry, and minor surgery. He or she performs the following services for patients:

1. Assessment of their total needs before these are categorized by specialty.

2. Elaboration of a plan for meeting those needs in the order of their importance.

3. Determination of who shall meet the defined needs - physicians, general or specialist; nonphysician members of the health team; or social agencies.

24. Although none of these careers would exactly correspond to your plans, which
    one most nearly corresponds to the 1st choice career you <u>plan</u> to follow?

    <u>First</u> choice career number _____

    Which career would be your <u>second</u> choice? _____   (6-8)

    Which career would you <u>least</u> like to pursue? _____

25. How certain are you that you will follow through on this <u>planned</u>
    career? (Check one)

    Very certain _____ 1

    Certain _____ ,2   (9)

    Doubtful _____ 3

26. Is there a career which you prefer to the one you ranked as your
    Number 1 planned career in question 24? (Check one)

    Yes _____ 1

    No _____ 2   (10)

27. Rank the following factors in order of their importance in the choice of
    your career by writing "1" for the most important, "2" for the next in
    importance, and so on.

    Rank assigned

    Intellectual content of the career   _____
    Example of a physician in this career   _____
    Social factors, such as colleagues,   _____   (11-15)
        type of patient, etc.   _____
    Working hours   _____
    Other   _____
        What?_____

SPECIALTY CHOICE

28. Even though you may not have arrived at a definite choice for your planned specialty, place a "1" next to your first choice, a "2" next to your second choice, and an "X" next to the specialty in which you would least like to work (DO NOT RANK ALL ITEMS).

Medicine, general	_____	1
Medicine, subspecialty		
Allergy and immunology	_____	2
Cardiology	_____	3
Gastroenterology	_____	4
Pulmonary diseases	_____	5
Other medical sub-		
specialty, what?_____		6
Surgery, general		7
Surgery, subspecialty		
Abdominal	_____	8
Neurosurgery	_____	
Orthopedic surgery	_____	10
Plastic surgery	_____	11
Thoracic surgery	_____	12
Urology	_____	13
Other surgical sub-		
specialty, what?_____		14
Other specialties		
Anesthesiology	_____	15
Basic scientist	_____	16
Dermatology	_____	17
Family (General		(16-17)
practice)	_____	18
Nuclear medicine	_____	19
Obstetrics and		
gynecology	_____	20
Ophthalmology	_____	21
Otolaryngology	_____	22
Pathology	_____	23
Pediatrics (General)	_____	24
Pediatrics subspecialty		
Allergist	_____	25
Cardiologist	_____	26
Physical medicine and		
rehabilitation	_____	27
Public Health:		
Bacterial	_____	28
Environmental	_____	29
Health care delivery	_____	30
Psychiatry	_____	31
Neurology	_____	32
Radiology	_____	33
Other - What?_____		34

MODE OF WORK

29. Even though you may not have arrived at a definite choice for your planned mode of work, place a "1" next to your first choice, and a "2" next to your second choice (DO NOT RANK ALL ITEMS - RANK ONLY 2 ITEMS)

Full time medical school faculty	_____ 1
Part time medical school faculty; part time private practice solo, or part time practice group	_____ 2
Full time private practice solo or group, with no medical school affiliation	_____ 3
Full time government employee	_____ 4
Part time government employee; part time medical school	_____ 5
Part time government employee; part time private practice, solo or group	_____ 6
Don't know	_____ 7
Other - what?	_____ 8

(18-20)

IN THE ABOVE LIST, PLACE AN "X" NEXT TO THE MODE OF WORK YOU WOULD LEAST LIKE TO FOLLOW.

30. In your career, where do you plan to derive <u>MOST</u> of your <u>INCOME</u>?
    (Check one)

Solo practice, fee for service	___ 1
Group practice fee for service	___ 2
Group practice, monthly prepaid	___ 3
Medical school employment	___ 4
Hospital employment	___ 5
Government employment	___ 6

    (21)

31. How do you expect to obtain most of your patients? (Check one)

Referred by other doctors	___ 1
By being selected by the patient	___ 2
Assigned by rotation in a group or hospital practice	___ 3

    (22)

<u>PLACE OF WORK</u>

32. It is now possible, whether you are in private practice or academic
    medicine, to choose the location of your work with patients. <u>Rank</u>
    order <u>all</u> of the following in order of your preference, from "1" --
    most preferred -- to "7" -- least preferred.

	Rank assigned
Ghetto	_____
Rural	_____
Suburban	_____
Urban-non-ghetto	_____
Foreign country	_____
Indian reservation	_____
Military service	_____

    (23-29)

33. Are there any discrepancies between the location you would <u>LIKE</u> to work
    and the location you <u>EXPECT</u> to work? (Check one)

Yes	___ 1
No	___ 2

    (30)

If the answer is <u>yes</u>, please explain the discrepancies._____

_____

_____

34. What percentage of your time do you plan to work in the following
    areas? (Amounts should total 100%)

	Percent	
Ghetto	_____	(31-33)
Rural	_____	(34-36)
Suburban	_____	(37-39)
Urban, no-ghetto	_____	(40-42)
Foreign country	_____	(43-45)
Indian Reservation	_____	(46-48)
Military service	_____	(49-51)
Total	100%	

TIME ALLOTMENT

35. As a physician, approximately what percentage of time would you ideally
    <u>LIKE</u> to spend in each of the following professional activities?
    (Amounts should total 100%)

	Percent	
Research	_____	(52-54)
Taking care of patients	_____	(55-57)
Administration	_____	(58-60)
Teaching	_____	(61-63)
Total	100%	

36. Approximately what percentage of your time do you <u>EXPECT</u> to spend in the following activities? (Amounts should total 100%)

	Percent	
Research	_____	(64-66)
Taking care of patients	_____	(67-69)
Administration	_____	(70-72)
Teaching	_____	(73-75)
Total	100%	

37. Are there any discrepancies between how you would <u>LIKE</u> to spend your time and how you <u>EXPECT</u> to spend your time? (Check one)

Yes _____ 1

No _____ 2

(76)

If the answer is <u>yes</u>, please explain the discrepancies:_____

_____

_____

Col. 80-2

38. Of the time that you <u>EXPECT</u> to spend in taking care of patients, approximately what percentage of this time would be devoted to the following: (Amounts should total 100%)

	Percent	
Hospitalized patients	_____	(6-8)
Ambulatory care of patients previously hospitalized	_____	(9-11)
Office care of patients, not hospitalized but requiring the care of a specialist	_____	(12-14)
Primary care, day-to-day care of illnesses which could also be treated by a family (general) practitioner i.e. first patient contact practice	_____	(15-17)
Total	100%	

39. In your career, where do you plan to spend <u>MOST</u> of your <u>TIME</u>?
    (Check one)

Solo practice, fee for service	_____1	
Group practice, fee for service	_____2	
Group practice, monthly prepaid	_____3	
Medical school faculty	_____4	(18)
Hospital employment	_____5	
Government employment	_____6	

40. Twenty years from now, how many hours per week...

    Do you <u>EXPECT</u> to work professionally? (Check one)

20-30 hrs.	_____1	
31-40 hrs.	_____2	
41-50 hrs.	_____3	(19)
51-60 hrs.	_____4	
Over 61 hrs.	_____5	

    Would you <u>LIKE</u> to work professionally? (Check one)

20-30 hrs.	_____1	
31-40 hrs.	_____2	
41-50 hrs.	_____3	(20)
51-60 hrs.	_____4	
Over 61 hrs.	_____5	

41. If there is a discrepancy between the number of hours you expect to
    work professionally and the number you would like to work, do you feel
    that this will be because of: (Check as many as you feel appropriate)

a.	Family needs	_____	(21)
b.	Availability of opportunities to do what you would like to do outside of medicine	_____	(22)
c.	Pressure from demands of practice	_____	(23)
d.	Competitive pressures derived from wish for advancement	_____	(24)
e.	Other	_____	(25)

  What? _____

  _____

GENERAL

42. Which phase of your medical training do you think will be the most important for your later career in medicine? (Check one)

First two years of medical school_____1
Last two years of medical school _____2
Internship _____3   (26)
Residency _____4
Don't know _____5

43. At the present time, do you have any doubts about medicine as a career for you? (Check one)

Yes, serious doubts _____1
Yes, slight doubts _____2   (27)
A few doubts _____3
No doubts at all _____4

44. Have you had doubts about whether you wished an M.D or a PhD? (Check one)

Yes, serious doubts _____1
Yes, slight doubts _____2   (28)
A few doubts _____3
No doubts at all _____4

45. Do you NOW have doubts about whether you wish an M.D. or a PhD? (Check one)

Yes, serious doubts _____1
Yes, slight doubts _____2   (29)
A few doubts _____3
No doubts at all _____4

46. Have you or do you plan to get a Phd? (Check one)

Yes _____1   (30)
No _____2

47. On which activities are you interested in spending time <u>after</u> graduation
from medical school? <u>Rank</u> them in order of their importance by
writing "1" for the most important, "2" for the next in importance,
<u>and so on for each activity on the list.</u> (Rank <u>all</u> 6 items.)

	Rank assigned	
Career or occupation	____	(31)
Leisure-time recreational activities	____	(32)
Participation as citizen in affairs of own community	____	(33)
Family relationships	____	(34)
Religious beliefs or activities	____	(35)
Activities directed toward national or international betterment	____	(36)

48. After you have completed your residency training, which of the
following will be your means of keeping up with advances in
medicine? (Express your answer in terms of a <u>percentage</u>, including
the "Other – What?" category if it applies: (Amounts should total
100%)

	Percent	
Reading journals and books	____ %	(37-39)
Attending medical meetings	____ %	(40-42)
Taking post-graduate course	____ %	(43-45)
Hospital rounds	____ %	(46-48)
Other – What? _____	____ %	(49-51)

_____

_____

49. <u>Rank</u> the following men in order from the person most admired, "1", to the
person least admired, "3".

	Rank	
Churchill	____	(52)
Pasteur	____	(53)
Freud	____	(54)

50. What are your reactions -- negative, neutral or positive -- to the following types of patients? (Check <u>one</u> for <u>each</u> type of Patient)

	Negative	Neutral	Positive	
Children	1	2	3	(55)
Young people	1	2	3	(56)
People with terminal illnesses	1	2	3	(57)
People who have psychogenic symptoms	1	2	3	(58)
Old people	1	2	3	(59)
People who have clearcut physical illnesses	1	2	3	(60)
Poor people	1	2	3	(61)
Rich people	1	2	3	(62)
The worried well	1	2	3	(63)

FINANCING YOUR MEDICAL EDUCATION

51. How difficult will it be for you to finance your medical education? (Check one)

Very difficult _____1

Fairly difficult _____2

Not very difficult _____3   (64)

Not at all difficult_____4

52. Are you a resident of the state in which your medical school is located? (Check one)

Yes_____

No_____   (65)

Col. 80-3

52. What percentage of your medical education expenses do you plan to receive from the following sources? (The amounts should total 100%)

Parents_____%	(6-8)
Spouse_____%	(9-11)
Other relatives_____%	(12-14)
Scholarship_____%	(15-17)
Loans_____%	(18-20)
Personal Earnings_____%	(21-23)
GI Bill of Rights_____%	(24-26)
Armed Services or Public Health Services_____%	(27-29)

Total 100%

53. Do you expect to receive any scholarship aid for your medical education? (Check one)

Yes_____1

No_____2   (30)

54. Upon graduation, do you expect to owe money for your medical education? (Check one)

Yes_____1

No_____2   (31)

If YES, approximately how much will you owe?
(Check one)

Less than $1000_____1

$1000-$2000_____2

$2000-$5000_____3   (32)

$5000-$10000_____4

$10000-$15000_____5

More than $15000_____6

55. What things do you think you will like best about being a doctor? (Check
    one category on each line)

	Like to a very great extent	Like to a great extent	Like to some extent	Like to a little extent	Like to a very little extent	
Being able to deal directly with people	1	2	3	4	5	(33)
Being able to help other people	1	2	3	4	5	(34)
The fact that medicine is a highly respected profession	1	2	3	4	5	(35)
Having interesting and intelligent people for colleagues	1	2	3	4	5	(36)
Doing work involving scientific method	1	2	3	4	5	(37)
Being my own boss	1	2	3	4	5	(38)
Being sure of earning an excellent income	1	2	3	4	5	(39)
The challenging and stimulating nature of the work	1	2	3	4	5	(40)
Using medicine to change society or the social system	1	2	3	4	5	(41)
Dealing with the psychological problems of patients	1	2	3	4	5	(42)
Ability to combine working with people with research	1	2	3	4	5	(43)
The fact that, within medicine, if certain career patterns are followed an individual can attain great prestige and status	1	2	3	4	5	(44)

56. A physician can be of service to his patients in a number of ways. <u>Rank</u> order the importance you attach to the following with a "1" for "most important" to a "3" for "least important." Rank <u>all</u> three items on the list.

	Rank Assigned	
Doing research on the problems of disease	_____	(45)
Treating patients directly	_____	(46)
Preventive medicine	_____	(47)

57. Do you plan to be politically active with respect to questions of health on the community and/or national level? (Check one)

Yes _____ 1
No _____ 2   (48)

58. In the running of a Neighborhood Clinic, which of the following administrative arrangements do you prefer? Policy is decided by: (Check one)

Representatives of the community; the physicians carry them out _____ 1

The community and the physicians on an equal basis _____ 2   (49)

The physicians, after consultation with the community _____ 3

59. In securing changes in the delivery of medical care to the community, which do you favor? (Check one)

Action without careful analysis and research, but evaluation afterwards making changes as necessary _____ 1

Careful analysis and research before action _____ 2   (50)

60. Do you plan to be politically active in other social issues on the community and/or national level? (Check one)

Yes _____ 1
No _____ 2   (51)

61. Do you think "fee for service" should be retained for the majority of physicians? (Check one)

                                        Yes_____1
                                        No_____2 (52)

                    For yourself?   (Check one)

                                        Yes_____1
                                        No_____2 (53)

62. Do you think the majority of physicians should be in group practice or solo practice? (Check one)

                                        Group_____1
                                        Solo_____2 (54)

        Which do you prefer for yourself?   (Check one)

                                        Group_____1
                                        Solo_____2 (55)

            If you prefer a group practice for yourself, do you favor a multi-specialist group or a uni-specialist group? (Check one)

                                    Multi-specialist_____1
                                    Uni-specialist_____2 (56)

63. If you prefer a group practice, how important are each of the following for your choice of group practice? Give each a percentage with all totaling 100%.

        A group would enable me to control my hours of work, so that the increased efficiency, coupled with much less night work, would allow me to spend more time with my family and on other activities outside of medicine.   _____% (57-59)

        Increase the level of competency of the practice of medicine, since a group of physicians with varied training can give a higher level of care, than one physician who does all things.   _____% (60-62)

        The pooling of office expenses thus lowering the costs of practice and making possible laboratory and x-ray facilities as well as allied health personnel, which would not be possible in solo practice.   _____% (63-65)

                                    Total: 100%

64. For your internship, which type of hospital would you choose: (Check one)

    A. Highly specialized hospital   _____ 1
    B. Out-patient Community
        Oriented Hospital   _____ 2 (66)

65. Ten years from now, when you are launched in your career, which type of hospital would you prefer to be affiliated with: (Check one)

    A. Highly specialized hospital   _____ 1
    B. Out-patient Community
        Oriented Hospital   _____ 2 (67)

66. Would you like to work on a full-time basis for the government? (Check one)

    Yes _____ 1 (68)
    No _____ 2

67. In your practice would you utilize the following assistants? (Check any you <u>would</u> use)

High school graduate with two years specialized training	_____	(69)
Nurse with additional two years training	_____	(70)
College graduate with a Baccalaureate Degree educated as a doctor's assistant	_____	(71)
Two-Year Junior College graduate trained as a doctor's assistant	_____	(72)
Discharged Navy Corpsmen	_____	(73)

68. Would you utilize paramedical personnel in the following areas? (Check the areas if you <u>would</u> utilize the personnel)

Minor surgery	_____	(74)
Well-baby clinic	_____	(75)
Handling emotional, social and family aspects of patients with physical problems	_____	(76)
Diagnosis and treatment of minor illnesses	_____	(77)

Col. 80-4

69. <u>Rank</u> order the importance to you of the following areas of social
    responsibility by writing "1" for the most important, "2" for the next in
    importance, <u>and so on for each statement</u>. Rank <u>all five</u> statements.

                                                              Rank Assigned

      Attention to the emotional, social, and
      family aspects of the care of patients;
      i.e., The Art of Medicine   ____   (6)

      Technological and scientific competence
      of a physician   ____   (7)

      Delivery of optimal care to all segments
      of the population without regard to
      finances   ____   (8)

      Research   ____   (9)

      A Preventive Medicine which takes
      action on the social factors which
      cause disease and which impedes health   ____   (10)

70. In his concern with the social factors, such as housing, education, hunger,
    etc., which impede health and produce disease, should the physician's prime
    effort be: (Check the <u>one</u> most important to you)

      To change these factors through political action
      with the community   ____ 1

      To develop with the community, neighborhood clinics
      and Public Health programs aimed at finding people
      who are ill and making modern care available to
      them   ____ 2   (11)

      The physician should not be concerned with social
      factors   ____ 3

71. Have the cuts in research funds affected your career choice? (Check one)

                              Yes ____ 1 (12)
                              No ____ 2

      If the answer is "Yes", in what way? _____

      _____

      _____

      _____

72. Are you in favor of the states requiring each physician to take an examination for relicensure every six years? (Check one)

Yes _____ 1   (13)
No _____ 2

73. Which of the following do you esteem most highly? <u>Rank</u> them from the highest "1", to the lowest "3". Rank <u>all three</u> items.

<u>Rank Assigned</u>

Intellectual tasks _____ (14)
Interpersonal relationships _____ (15)
Introspection _____ (16)

74. Were you on a varsity athletic team in college? (Check one)

Yes _____ 1   (17)
No _____ 2

75. Regardless of whether you were on a varsity team, rate your athletic ability (Check one)

Excellent _____ 1
Good _____ 2   (18)
Fair _____ 3
Poor _____ 4

76. Do you like to work with your hands? (Check one)

Very much _____ 1
Some _____ 2   (19)
Little _____ 3

77. How skillful are you in doing mechanical work? (Check one)

Excellent _____ 1
Good _____ 2   (20)
Fair _____ 3
Poor _____ 4

78. Which of the following most accurately describes the type of physician you wish to become? (Check one)

> Primarily a scientist, who helps people
> by treating their illnesses using a
> high level of scientific knowledge   1
>
> Primarily interested in working directly
> with people, being of service to them,   (21)
> treating their illnesses using science
> pragmatically   2

79. Many have stated that for high scientific achievement, competition must be stimulated in order that the most able students academically emerge to do science and secure the research grants. On the other hand, it is stated that the delivery of medical care requires the development of cooperative physicians who can work well with other physicians, health workers, patients and communities. These two views of physicians are the antithesis of each other. They can be placed at the two ends of a continuum as competitive versus cooperative. Where would you place yourself on this continuum?

> Very competitive   1
> Very competitive, somewhat cooperative   2
> Equally competitive and cooperative   3   (22)
> Somewhat competitive, very cooperative   4
> Very cooperative   5

80. How much do you expect to earn, twenty years from now, keeping the value of the dollar constant, i.e., at today's prices:

> Less than $20,000   1
> 20,000 to 30,000   2
> 30,000 to 40,000   3   (23)
> 40,000 to 50,000   4
> 50,000 to 75,000   5
> more than 75,000   6

81. Are you in favor in medical school of a letter or numerical grading system, or a Pass-Fail system? (Check one)

> Letter or numerical
> Grading System   1
> Pass-Fail   2   (24)

CARE IN SCARCITY AREAS

82. Would you be in favor of a National Service Corps for physicians, in which every physician, male or female, would have to serve one or two years in a medically deprived area in order to obtain a permanent license? (Check one)

Yes_____ 1
No_____ 2   (25)

83. Would you work in a medical institution such as a hospital or a clinic, in which the consumers are the majority of the governing board? (Check one)

Yes_____ 1
No_____ 2   (26)

84. Who do you feel should set physicians fees? (Check one)

Physicians_____ 1
Consumer groups_____ 2   (27)
Bargaining between the two groups _____ 3
                                        2

85. A proposal has been made for a National Health Insurance Plan in which each person able to pay has a certain amount added to his annual income tax; the government pays for those unable to pay; and the government uses these funds to pay for medical care. Are you in favor of such a plan?

Yes_____ 1
No_____ 2   (28)

86. If a National Health Insurance Plan is passed by Congress, do you think it should: (Check one)

Include the total population? _____ 1
Include only those too poor to purchase
    services themselves? _____ 2   (29)

87. Should a National Health Insurance Plan: (Check one)

Give funds to the consumer to pay
    services? _____ 1
Regulate the use of funds so that the
    system for the delivery of health
    care is changed? _____ 2   (30)

88. Which do you think will be the prevailing mode of medical practice in
    1985? (Check one)

     Solo practice, fee for service _____ 1
     Group practice, fee for service _____ 2 (31)
     Group practice, monthly pre-payment plan _____ 3
     All physicians employed by the government _____ 4

89. Check one of the following:

     1. I plan to practice in a medically deprived area
        regardless of any supportive programs _____ 1

     2. No combination of supportive programs would
        convince me to practice in a medically
        deprived area. _____ 2 (32)

     3. I would practice in a medically deprived area
        if certain supportive programs were available _____ 3

90. If you checked 3 in the above question, indicate the importance of <u>each</u>
    of the following supportive programs, as an incentive for <u>you</u> to practice
    in a medically deprived area. (1) would indicate it is of great importance
    to you, (4) that it is of little importance to you. (Check one category
    on each line.)

	1	2	3	4	
Not having to pay back the loans for my medical education.	_____	_____	_____	_____	(33)
Scholarship for all expenses in medical school.	_____	_____	_____	_____	(34)
Membership in a group practice.	_____	_____	_____	_____	(35)
Medical school appointment.	_____	_____	_____	_____	(36)
Large annual income.	_____	_____	_____	_____	(37)

91. Indicate the importance of <u>each</u> of the following supportive programs as an incentive for all physicians, not necessarily you, to practice in a medically deprived area. "1" would indicate that it is of great importance, "4" that it is of little importance. (Check one category on each line.)

	1	2	3	4	
Not having to pay back the loans for medical education.	____	____	____	____	(38)
Scholarship for all expenses in medical school.	____	____	____	____	(39)
Membership in a group practice.	____	____	____	____	(40)
Medical school appointment.	____	____	____	____	(41)
Large annual income.	____	____	____	____	(42)

92. How much will your career be affected by the following? (Check <u>one</u> category on each line.)

	1 None	2 Slightly	3 Moderately	4 Greatly	
Economic Factors:	____	____	____	____	(43)
Social Factors:	____	____	____	____	(44)
Other:	____	____	____	____	(45)

What?_____

93. There is great difficulty in defining "family practice". Do you consider that you will be primarily a family practitioner?

Yes _____ 1
No _____ 2   (46)

If the answer is "Yes", what will be the vehicle? (Check one)

General internal medicine _____ 1
General pediatrics _____ 2
General practice _____ 3   (47)
Other, what? _____ 4

94. In which direction do you think medical school admissions policies should be changed? To admit ... (Check one)

More scientifically oriented students_____1

More people oriented students_____2   (48)

95. Rank order the priorities that medical school admission policy should give to admitting more of the following students. "1" would indicate the highest priority, "3" the lowest.

<u>Rank assigned</u>

Scientifically oriented _____   (49)
Interpersonally oriented _____   (50)
Psychologically oriented _____   (51)

96. Do you consider yourself primarily: (Check one)

Scientifically oriented_____1
Interpersonally oriented_____2   (52)
Psychologically oriented_____3

97. Do you think that medical schools should have two curricula: a bioscientific one for the eduction of academicians and sub-specialists, the other a biosocial one for the eduction of family practitioners, public health physicians, and psychiatrists? (Check one)

Yes_____1

No_____2   (53)

98. Many think that a primary issue in medicine is the depersonalization and dehumanization of patient care. Do you agree? (Check one)

Yes_____1

No_____2   (54)

If your answer is YES, how would you change this? _____

_____

_____

99. How much of a part should other professional medical people such as Hospital Administrators, Nurses, Social Workers, etc., have in the decisions relating to medical care delivery? (Check one)

Less than physicians _____	1	
Equal to physicians _____	2	(55)
More than physicians _____	3	

100. How much of a part should these other professional medical people have in the decisions concerning individual patient care? (Check one).

Less than the physician _____	1	
Equal to the physician _____	2	(56)
More than the physician _____	3	

101. Should a National Health Insurance Plan allow for enrollment on a: (Check one)

Voluntary basis _____	1	
Compulsory basis _____	2	(57)

102. Are you a transfer student from another medical school? (Check one)

Yes _____	1	
No _____	2	(58)

If yes, from what school? _____

103. Name the colleges where you received your Pre Medical Education?

_____   (59)

104. Are you dissatisfied with the present method of health care delivery? (Check one)

                    Yes_____

                    No_____   (60)

105. Who do you think are the most important persons in medicine at the present time?

            _____ (61)

106. The infant and maternal mortality rate is much higher in the slums than in the suburbs. If you were appointed as a one person commission by the mayor of a large city and were given unlimited funds to solve this problem, outline how you would proceed:

    _____

    _____

    _____

    _____   (62)

    _____

    _____

    _____

107. Do you think the current system of medical care delivery is: (Check one)

                    Very satisfactory_____1

                         Satisfactory_____2 (63)

                      Unsatisfactory_____3

              Very unsatisfactory_____4

108. If National Health Insurance is passed:

    a. Should it provide funds for only a certain number of physicians in a specialty to practice in any one geographical area, thus making up for the current maldistribution of physicians throughout the various geographical areas in the U.S.? (Check one)

                    Yes_____1 (64)

                    No_____2

    b. Should it only fund a certain number of physicians practicing in any specialty, thus forcing a redistribution of physicians in the specialties according to the perceived needs of society? (Check one)

                    Yes_____1 (65)

                    No_____2

                              Col. 80-5

4. Listed below are **six** (6) proposals currently under consideration by the new Congress. If such legislation is inevitable, which alternatives, if any, do you:

> 1) favor strongly.
> 2) find acceptable, <u>even if disagreeable</u>.
> 3) find so unacceptable that you would not have applied to medical school had it been already instituted.

National service agreements must be secured from: (Check one on each line)

	Agree	Acceptable	Unacceptable	
a. All entering students, using a lottery to select those graduates needed to serve	___1	___2	___3	(10)
b. 25% of entering students - with each student being given substantial federal support for tuition and living expenses	___1	___2	___3	(11)
c. All entering students - with <u>all</u> being given such federal support and all being required to serve	___1	___2	___3	(12)
d. All entering students, all of whom must serve unless they reimburse the government for capitation payments (presently $2100 per student per year) - <u>in addition to</u> paying tuition	___1	___2	___3	(13)
e. All students who receive financial aid	___1	___2	___3	14)
f. Medical schools should be free - with all physicians employed by a National Health Service	___1	___2	___3	(15)

5. If national service agreements are required by law, should the medical schools be liable for loss of federal funds if a student defaults on his/her agreement? (Check one)

Yes____1
No____2 (16)

6. Is present U.S. reliance on practicing foreign medical graduates an undesirable situation? (Check one)

Yes____1
No____2 (17)

HEALTH MANPOWER LEGISLATION POLL

1. Health manpower bills in different forms were passed by BOTH HOUSE AND
SENATE during the last session.

2. In the present Congress, these bills have been reintroduced and the debate
will begin anew. Knowledgeable observers predict that <u>some</u> form of
health manpower legislation is virtually inevitable.

These bills attempt to splve these current problems in American Medicine:

   1. Geographic and specialty maldistribution of physicians.

   2. Dependence on foreign medical graduates. (FMG's)

Please answer the following questions concerning these important matters.

1.   Is it the responsibility of the federal government to insure that solutions
are found to major health caré delivery problems? (Check one)

Yes_____1
No_____2   (6)

2.   Are you opposed to <u>any</u> form of mandatory service - even if voluntary
federal programs using financial incentives to encourage practice in
underserved areas prove extremely expensive to the taxpayer? (Check one)

Yes_____1   (7)
No_____2

3. Would you:

   a. Continue to support "no strings attached" aid to
      medical education? (Check one)

Yes_____1   (8)
No_____2

   b. Accept the inevitability of conditions on aid and seek
      to limit them to ones to which most schools could respond
      and which meet national goals? (Check one)

Yes_____1   (9)
No_____2

7. Should there be a reduction in the number of first year residency training slots to 125% of the U.S. medical schools graduates in order to reduce the number of FMG's? (Check one)

Yes_____1

No_____2   (18)

8. Should there be control over the distribution of first year residency training slots among the various specialties in order to increase the proportion devoted to preparation of primary care physicians? (Check one)

Yes_____1

No_____2   (19)

9. Should there be control over the geographical location of first year residency training slots as one means to insure adequate distribution of physicians after training? (Check one)

Yes_____1

No_____2   (20)

10. If your answer to question 7, 8, or 9 was "Yes", would you prefer that control be exercised by: (Check one)

   a. A federal commission whose members would
      be appointed by the HEW Secretary   _____1

   b. The private sector, through a non-govern-   (21)
      ment group such as the Coordinating
      Council on Medical Education   _____

11. Approximately, what was your GPA in:

   a. Science courses: _____   (22-24)

   b. Non-science courses: _____   (25-27)

Col. 80-6

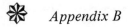 *Appendix B*

Physician's Questionnaire

NAME_____

MEDICAL SCHOOL _____ (6)

TODAY'S DATE_____

YEAR OF GRADUATION FROM MEDICAL SCHOOL   _____ (7-8)

SEX (Check one)   Male_____1
                                                   Female_____2 (9)

1. Your father's occupation? Be specific. (If retired or deceased, please
   indicate his former occupation.)
   _____ (10)

2. Your father's education? (Circle highest level attained)
   GRADE SCHOOL   HIGH SCHOOL   COLLEGE   POST-GRADUATE
   1 2 3 4 5 6 7 8   9 10 11 12   13 14 15 16   17 18 19 20 and over   (11-12)

3. Your mother's education? (Circle highest level attained)
   GRADE SCHOOL   HIGH SCHOOL   COLLEGE   POST-GRADUATE
   1 2 3 4 5 6 7 8   9 10 11 12   13 14 15 16   17 18 19 20 and over   (13-14)

4. Your mother's occupation? Be specific. If Housewife, check here _____
   _____ (15)

165

5. Which of the following best describes the place where you grew up?
    (Check one)

A farm or ranch	_____	1	
A town of less than 10,000	_____	2	
A small city of from 10,000 to 100,000	_____	3	(16)
A suburb of a large city	_____	4	
Within a large city	_____	5	
You moved so much it would be hard to say	_____	6	

6. Is or was your mother or father a doctor?

Neither	_____	1	
Mother	_____	2	(17)
Father	_____	3	
Both	_____	4	

7. Did you ever interrupt your undergraduate college education for a year or
    more? (Check one)

Yes	_____	1	(18)
No	_____	2	

8. Indicate how many summers you worked in the following areas before
    medical school:

Hospital work with patients	_____	
Lab assistant or technician in a hospital	_____	(19-22)
Research	_____	
Work in slums or rural areas	_____	

9. How many summers was it necessary for you to earn money to support
    yourself as an undergraduate in college?

none	_____	0	
1	_____	1	
2	_____	2	(23)
3	_____	3	
4	_____	4	

...in medical school?

none	_____	0	
1	_____	1	
2	_____	2	(24)
3	_____	3	
4	_____	4	

10. Did you have to work to support yourself during the academic year as an undergraduate at college (excluding summers)?

Yes ——— 1 (25)
No ——— 2

...in medical school?

Yes ——— 1 (26)
No ——— 2

11. From which type of secondary school were you graduated? (Check one)

Public ——— 1 (27)
Private ——— 2
Parochial ——— 3

12. <u>Rank</u> the following subjects according to the amount of pleasure they gave you during college by writing "1" for the most enjoyable subject, <u>and so on</u> to "4" for the least enjoyable subject.

Rank assigned

Natural sciences ————————
Behavioral sciences ———————— (28-31)
Humanities ————————
Social sciences ————————

13. Did you do any research while an undergraduate at college?

Yes ——— 1 (32)
No ——— 2

...in medical school?

Yes ——— 1 (33)
No ——— 2

14. If you did any research during college, specify which field: (Check the predominant field)

Biology	_____	1	
Chemistry	_____	2	
Biochemistry	_____	3	
Physics	_____	4	
Public Health	_____	5	(34)
Social Sciences	_____	6	
Behavioral Sciences	_____	7	
Other	_____	8	
What?	_____		

...in medical school:

Basic Sciences	_____	1	
Clinical Sciences	_____	2	
Psychiatry	_____	3	(35)
Public Health	_____	4	
Other (specify)	_____	5	

15. Rank the following subjects according to the grades you received in them in college by writing "1" for the highest grades, "2" for the next, and so on to "4".

	Rank assigned	
Natural sciences	_____	
Behavioral sciences	_____	
Humanities	_____	(36-39)
Social sciences	_____	

16. Before deciding on medicine, did you ever seriously consider any other occupation or profession?

Yes _____ 1 (40)
No _____ 2

If yes, did you ever seriously consider a career in one or more of the following fields? (Check as many as apply)

Sciences, PhD level	_____
Humanities, PhD level	_____
Social Sciences, PhD level	_____
Psychology, PhD level	_____
Becoming a businessman or woman	_____
Becoming a lawyer	_____
Becoming a teacher of elementary or secondary school	_____ (41-53)
Becoming a Social Worker	_____
Going to a School of Public Health	_____
Becoming a Hospital Administrator	_____
Becoming an Engineer	_____
Becoming an Architech	_____
Other, What? _____	

17. Did you have difficulty in making up your mind whether to pursue an M.D. or PhD?

Yes _____ 1 (54)
No _____ 2

If yes, which of the following areas did you consider for a PhD? (Check one)

Natural sciences	_____	1
Behavioral sciences	_____	2 (55)
Humanities	_____	3
Social sciences	_____	4

18. If on several attempts, you had failed to secure entrance to any medical school would you have: (Check one)

Gone to graduate schools in the natural sciences	_____	1
Gone to graduate school in the humanities	_____	2
Gone to graduate school in the social sciences	_____	3
Gone to graduate school in psychology	_____	4
Become a businessman	_____	5
Become a lawyer	_____	6
Become a teacher of elementary or secondary school	_____	7
Gone to Dental School	_____	8
Gone to Social Work School	_____	9
Gone to a School of Public Health	_____	10
Become a Hospital Administrator	_____	11
Become an Engineer or Architect	_____	12
Other, What?	_____	13

(56-57)

19. When did you <u>first</u> think of becoming a physician? (Check one)

Before college	_____	1
First two years of college	_____	2
Junior year	_____	3
Senior year	_____	4
After college	_____	5

(58)

20. When did you <u>consolidate</u> your career plans to become a physician? (Check one)

Before college	_____	1
First two years of college	_____	2
Junior year	_____	3
Senior year	_____	4
After college	_____	5

(59)

21. What was your college major or field of concentration? (Check one)

Biochemical Sciences	_____ 1
Biochemistry	_____ 2
Biology	_____ 3
Biophysics	_____ 4
Chemistry	_____ 5
Cultural Anthropology	_____ 6
Economics	_____ 7
Engineering	_____ 8 (60-61)
Government or Political Science	_____ 9
Humanities	_____ 10
Mathematics	_____ 11
Physics	_____ 12
Pre-Med	_____ 13
Psychology	_____ 14
Sociology	_____ 15

22. When you entered college did you plan to: (Check one)

Become a physician	_____ 1
Go to graduate school in the sciences	_____ 2
Go to graduate school in the humanities	_____ 3
Go to graduate school in the social sciences	_____ 4
Go to graduate school in psychology	_____ 5
Become a businessman	_____ 6
Become a lawyer	_____ 7
Become a teacher of elementary or secondary school	_____ 8 (62-63)
Go to dental school	_____ 9
Go to social work school	_____ 10
Go to a school of public health	_____ 11
Become a hospital administrator	_____ 12
Become an engineer or architect	_____ 13
Undecided	_____ 14
Other, What?	_____ 15
_____	

The following vignettes are descriptions of various careers of physicians. Please read them carefully since you will be asked to answer questions about the one which best corresponds to your present career.

CAREER NUMBER 1

This physician is a clinical Subspecialist. This doctor's education is basically bioscientific. If an internist, he or she is a cardiologist, gastroenterologist, allergist, etc. If a surgeon, an orthopedic surgeon, plastic surgeon, abdominal surgeon, neurosurgeon, etc. If in pediatrics, a pediatric cardiologist, a pediatric allergist, etc. If not in a subspecialty of a major specialty, he or she is in a specialty whose scope is narrowly defined. Examples of this would be neurology, pathology, radiology, etc.

CAREER NUMBER 2

This physician is a General Specialist. This doctor's education is basically bioscientific, but he or she is more interested in a broad range of problems within a specialty rather than a subspecialty. Examples of this are general internal medicine, general pediatrics, general surgery, etc.

CAREER NUMBER 3

This physician is a Basic Scientist. This doctor has no clinical practice, but is totally engaged in teaching and research in a basic science.

CAREER NUMBER 4

This physician is a Biomedical Engineer. This doctor majored in college in a physical science such as mathematics, computer science, engineering or physics and has a career dealing with medical problems which involve his or her knowledge of these sciences.

CAREER NUMBER 5

This physician is a Psychiatrist, primarily concerned with patients with psychological problems or mental illnesses.

CAREER NUMBER 6

This physician is a Public Health Physician. He or she not only has a medical education, but possibly also a degree in public health. This doctor deals directly with preventing diseases, research into their prevention, or into the problems of health care delivery, or administers either a hospital or community clinic.

CAREER NUMBER 7

This physician is a General Practitioner with the new name of Family Practitioner. He and she is engaged in diagnosis and treating not only patients' physical problems, but also the related family, social, and emotional aspects of the patients' illness. He or she has a broad training in internal medicine, pediatrics, minor surgery, and obstetrics and gynecology, and closely resembles the old style general practitioner.

23. Which career pattern most nearly corresponds to your present career?

Present career number   _____   (64)

24. Is there a career which you would prefer to your present career?

Yes   _____   1   (65)
No   _____   2

25. If there is a discrepancy between the career you are in and the career you prefer, please indicate the number of the career you prefer.

MY PREFERRED CAREER IS NUMBER   _____   (66)

If there is a discrepancy between the career you are in and the career you prefer, please explain why you are not following your preferred career:

_____

_____

_____

_____

26. Rank the following factors in order of their importance in the choice of your career by writing "1" for the most important, "2" for the next in importance, and so on. If any one or more of these factors are not important, omit them from the ranking.

Rank assigned

Intellectual content of the career   _____
Example of a physician in this career   _____
Social factors, such as colleagues,   (67-70)
   type of patient, etc.   _____
Working hours   _____

27. Is the career that you are following now the career you planned to follow when you graduated from medical school?

Yes _____ 1 (71)
No _____ 2

If the answer is NO, what is the number of the career you had planned?

Career Number _____ (72)

What caused you to change your career? _____

_____

_____

_____

28. Have you had any changes in career since you left medical school?

Yes _____ 1 (73)
No _____ 2

If YES, from Career Number _____ to Career Number _____

to Career Number _____

to Career Number _____   (74-78)

to Career Number _____

Please explain these changes _____

_____

_____

_____

_____

_____

_____

_____

Col. (80)-1

SPECIALTY CHOICE

29. Check your present specialty:

Medicine, general	_____	1
Medicine, subspecialty		
Allergy and immunology	_____	2
Cardiology	_____	3
Gastroenterology	_____	4
Pulmonary diseases	_____	5
Other medical sub- specialty, what?	_____	6
Surgery, general	_____	7
Surgery, subspecialty		
Abdominal	_____	8
Neurosurgery	_____	9
Orthopedic surgery	_____	10
Plastic surgery	_____	11
Thoracic surgery	_____	12
Urology	_____	13
Other surgical sub- specialty, what?	_____	14
Other specialties		
Anesthesiology	_____	15
Basic scientist	_____	16
Dermatology	_____	17
Family (General practice)	_____	18
Nuclear medicine	_____	19
Obstetrics and gyne- cology	_____	20
Opthamology	_____	21
Otolaryngology	_____	22
Pathology	_____	23
Pediatrics (General)	_____	24
Pediatrics subspecialty		
Allergist	_____	25
Cardiologist	_____	26
Physical medicine and rehabilitation	_____	27
Public Health:		
Bacterial	_____	28
Environmental	_____	29
Health care delivery	_____	30
Psychiatry	_____	31
Neurology	_____	32
Radiology	_____	33
Other - What?	_____	34

(6-7)
(8-15)

30. Are you certified in this specialty?   Yes _____ 1   (16)
                                                            No _____ 2

31. Is this the only specialty you have had since leaving medical school?

Yes ____ 1 (17)
No ____ 2

     If NO, go back to question #29 and place a "1" next to the specialty you were first in after medical school, a "2" in the next one, etc.

MODE OF WORK

32. Check the mode of work which you are now following:

                                  Full time medical school
faculty   ____ 1

                                    Part time medical school
faculty; part time private
practice solo, or part time
practice group, fee for
service   ____ 2

    Part time medical school
faculty; part time pre-
payment group   ____ 3

    Full time private practice   (18)
solo or group, with no
medical school affiliation   ____ 4 (19-22)

    Full time government
employee   ____ 5

    Part time government
employee; part time
medical school   ____ 6

    Part time government
employee; part time
private practice, solo
or group   ____ 7

    Other, what? _____ 8

33. Has this been your only mode of work since you completed your residency training?

Yes ____ 1 (23)
No ____ 2

     If NO, go back to question #32 and place a "1" next to the first mode of work you had after residency, a "2" after the next, a "3" after the next, etc.

34. Are you on the faculty of a medical school?

Yes _____ 1 (24)
No _____ 2

       If YES, what faculty rank?

Instructor _____ 1
Assistant Professor _____ 2 (25)
Associate Professor _____ 3
Professor _____ 4

35. How many years were you a house officer?

1 _____
2 _____
3 _____ (26)
4 _____
5 or more _____

36. How many years were you in a fellowship after medical school? _____ (27)

37. Do you have any degrees in addition to the Baccalaureate Degree and the M.D.?

Yes _____ 1 (28)
No _____ 2

      If so, what?

PhD _____ 1
MS or MA _____ 2 (29)
Other _____ 3

38. In your career, where do you derive MOST of your INCOME? (Check one)

Solo practice, fee for service _____ 1
Group practice fee for service _____ 2
Group practice, monthly prepaid _____ 3 (30)
Medical school employment _____ 4
Hospital employment _____ 5
Government employment _____ 6

39. How do you obtain most of your patients? (Check one)

Referral by other doctors _____ 1
By being selected by the patient _____ 2 (31)
Assigned by rotation in a group practice _____ 3

PLACE OF WORK

40. What percentage of your time do you work in the following areas?
(Amounts should total 100%)

	Percent	
Ghetto	_____	
Rural	_____	
Suburban	_____	
Urban, non-ghetto	_____	
Foreign country	_____	(32-52)
Indian Reservation	_____	
Military service	_____	
Total	100%	

TIME ALLOTMENT

41. Approximately what percentage of time do you spend in each of the
following professional activities? (Amounts should total 100%)

	Percent	
Research	_____	
Taking care of patients	_____	
Administration	_____	(53-64)
Teaching	_____	
Total	100%	

42. Approximately what percentage of your time would you PREFER to spend in
the following activities? (Amounts should total 100%)

	Percent	
Research	_____	
Taking care of patients	_____	
Administration	_____	(65-76)
Teaching	_____	
Total	100%	

Col (80) - 2

43. Are there any discrepencies between how you spend your time and how you would prefer to spend it?

                                                    Yes_____1
                                                    No_____2   (6)

    If there are any discrepencies, please explain them:_____

    _____

    _____

    _____

    _____

    _____

44. Of the time that you spend in taking care of patients, approximately what percentage of this time is devoted to the following? (Amounts should total 100%)

                                                              Percent

    Hospitalized patients   _____

    Ambulatory care of patients
    previously hospitalized   _____

    Office care of patients, not
    hospitalized but requiring
    the care of a specialist   _____

    Primary care, day-to-day care   (7-18)
    of illnesses which could also
    be treated by a family (general)
    practitioner i.e. first patient
    contact practice   _____

                                    Total   100%

45. In your career, what percentage of your time do you spend in each of the following areas? (Amounts should total 100%)

                                                              Percent

    Solo practice, fee for service _____

    Group practice, fee for service_____

    Group practice, monthly prepaid_____

    Medical school faculty   _____   (19-36)

    Hospital employment   _____

    Government employment   _____

                                    Total   100%

46. How many hours per week . . .

        Do you work professionally? (Check one)

20-30 hrs.	_____1	
31-40 hrs.	_____2	
41-50 hrs.	_____3	(37)
51-60 hrs.	_____4	
Over 61 hrs.	_____5	

        Would you <u>LIKE</u> to work professionally? (Check one)

20-30 hrs.	_____1	
31-40 hrs.	_____2	
41-50 hrs.	_____3	(38)
51-60 hrs.	_____4	
Over 61 hrs.	_____5	

47. If there is a discrepency between the number of hours you work and the number of hours you would like to work, do you feel that this is because of: (Check as many as you feel appropriate)

    a. Family needs   _____

    b. Availability of opportunities
        to do what you would like
        to do outside of medicine _____

    c. Pressure from demands of
        practice   _____   (39-43)

    d. Competitive pressures
        derived from wish for
        advancement   _____

    e. Other   _____

        What?_____

        _____

GENERAL

48. Which phase of your medical training do you think was the most important for your eventual career in medicine? (Check one)

First two years of medical school	_____	1
Last two years of medical school	_____	2
Internship	_____	3 (44)
Residency	_____	4
Don't know	_____	5

49. Rank the following men in order from the person most admired, "1", to to the person least admired, "3".

	Rank	
Churchill	_____	
Pasteur	_____	(45-47)
Freud	_____	

50. How difficult was it for you to finance your medical education? (Check one)

Very difficult	_____	1
Fairly difficult	_____	2 (48)
Not very difficult	_____	3
Not at all difficult	_____	4

51. What things do you like best about being a doctor? (Check <u>one</u> category
     on each line)

	Like to a very great extent	Like to a great extent	Like to some extent	Like to a little extent	Like to a very little extent
Being able to deal directly with people	1	2	3	4	5
Being able to help other people	1	2	3	4	5
The fact that medicine is a highly respected profession	1	2	3	4	5
Having interesting and intelligent people for colleagues	1	2	3	4	5
Doing work involving scientific method	1	2	3	4	5
Being my own boss	1	2	3	4	5
Being sure of earning an excellent income	1	2	3	4	5
The challenging and stimulating nature of the work	1	2	3	4	5
Using medicine to change society or the social system	1	2	3	4	5
Dealing with the psychological problems of patients	1	2	3	4	5
Ability to combine working with people with research	1	2	3	4	5
The fact that, within medicine, if certain career patterns are followed an individual can attain great prestige and status	1	2	3	4	5

(49-60)

52. A physician can be of service to his patients in a number of ways. <u>Rank</u> order the importance you attach to the following with a "1" for "most important" to a "3" for "least important." Rank <u>all</u> three items on the list.

<u>Rank Assigned</u>

Doing research on the
problems of disease   _____

Treating patients
directly   _____   (61-63)

Preventive medicine   _____

53. Are you politically active with respect to questions of health on the community and/or national level?   (Check one)

Yes _____ 1 (64)
No _____ 2

54. In the running of a Neighborhood Clinic, which of the following administrative arrangements do you prefer? Policy is decided by: (Check one)

Representatives of the community; the
physicians carry out the policy   _____ 1

The community and the physicians
on an equal basis   _____ 2 (65)

The physicians, after consultation
with the community   _____ 3

55. In securing changes in the delivery of medical care to the community, which do you favor? (Check one)

Action without careful analysis and
research, but evaluation afterwards
making changes as necessary   _____ 1
                                                        (66)
Careful analysis and research before
action   _____ 2

56. Do you think "fee for service" should be retained for the majority of physicians? (Check one)

Yes _____ 1 (67)
No _____ 2

For yourself? (Check one)

Yes _____ 1 (68)
No _____ 2

57. Do you think the majority of physicians should be in group practice or solo
     practice? (Check one)

                                                     Group _____ 1
                                                     Solo _____ 2 (69)

          Which are you in?

                                                     Group _____ 1
                                                     Solo _____ 2 (70)

          If you are in a group practice, is it a multi-specialist group
          or a uni-specialist group? (Check one)

                                         Multi-specialist _____ 1
                                         Uni-specialist   _____ 2 (71)

                                                     Col. (80)-3

58. If you are in a <u>group practice</u>, how important are each of the following
     for your choice of group practice? Give each a percentage with all
     totalling 100%.

                                                                <u>Percent</u>

          A group enables me to control my hours of work, so
          that the increased efficiency, coupled with much
          less night work, allows me to spend more time with
          my family and on other activities outside of
          medicine.   _____%

          A group increases the level of competency of the
          practice of medicine, since a group of physicians
          with varied training can give a higher level of
          care, than one physician who does all things.   _____%   (6-14)

          A group allows the pooling of office expenses thus
          lowering the costs of practice and making possible
          laboratory and x-ray facilities as well as allied
          health personnel, which would not be possible in
          solo practice.   _____%
                                             Total   100%

59. For your internship, which type of hospital did you choose? (Check one)

                                 A: Teaching Hospital   _____ 1
                                 B: Community Hospital   _____ 2 (15)
                                 C: Other, What? _____ 3

60. For your residency, which type of hospital did you choose? (Check one)

A: Teaching Hospital   _____   1
B: Community Hospital _____   2 (16)
C: Other, what? _____   3

61. Which type of hospital are you presently affiliated with? (Check the one you are most predominantly affiliated with)

A: Teaching Hospital   _____   1
B: Community Hospital _____   2 (17)
C: Other, what? _____   3

62. Would you like to work on a full-time basis for the government? (Check one)

Yes _____   1 (18)
No _____   2

63. In your practice, would you or do you utilize the following assistants? (Check any you would or do use)

High school graduate with two years specialized training   _____

Nurse with additional two years training   _____

College graduate with a Baccalaureate Degree educated as a doctor's assistant   _____   (19-23)

Two-Year Junior College graduate trained as a doctor's assistant   _____

Discharged Navy Corpsmen   _____

64. Would you or do you utilize paramedical personnel in the following areas? (Check the areas if you would or do utilize these personnel)

Minor surgery   _____

Well-baby clinic   _____

Handling emotional, social and family aspects of patients with physical problems   _____   (24-27)

Diagnosis and treatment of minor illnesses   _____

65. <u>Rank</u> order the importance to you of the following areas of social responsibility by writing "1" for the most important, "2" for the next in importance, <u>and so on for each statement</u>. Rank <u>all five</u> statements.

Rank Assigned

Attention to the emotional, social, and
family aspects of the care of patients;
i.e., The Art of Medicine

_____

Technological and scientific competence
of a physician

_____

Delivery of optimal care to all segments of
the population without regard to finances   _____   (28-32)

Research

_____

A Preventive Medicine which takes action
on the social factors which cause disease and
which impede health

_____

66. In his concern with the social factors, such as housing, education, hunger, etc., which impede health and produce disease, should the physician's prime effort be: (Check the <u>one</u> most important to you)

To change these factors through political action
within the community   _____ 1

To develop with the community, neighborhood clinics
and Public Health programs aimed at finding people
who are ill and making modern care available to   (33)
them   _____ 2

The physician should not be concerned with social
factors   ·   _____ 3

67. Have the cuts in federal funds for medicine affected your career? (Check one)

Yes   _____ 1 (34)
No   _____ 2

If the answer is "YES", in what way? _____

_____

_____

_____

_____

68. Are you in favor of the states requiring each physician to take an examination for relicensure every six years? (Check one)

Yes _____ 1
No _____ 2 (35)

69. Which of the following do you esteem most highly? <u>Rank</u> them from the highest "1", to the lowest "3". Rank <u>all three</u> items.

Rank Assigned

Intellectual tasks
Interpersonal relationships _____ (36-38)
Introspection

70. Which of the following most accurately describes the type of physician you are? (Check one)

A. Primarily a scientist, who helps people by treating their illnesses using a high level of scientific knowledge _____ 1

B. Primarily interested in working directly with people, being of service to them, (39) treating their illnesses using science pragmatically _____ 2

71. Many have stated that for high scientific achievement, competition must be stimulated in order that the most able students academically emerge to do science and secure the research grants. On the other hand, it is stated that the delivery of medical care requires the development of cooperative physicians who can work well with other physicians, health workers, patients and communities. These two views of physicians are the antithesis of each other. They can be placed at the two ends of a continuum as competitive versus cooperative. Where would you place yourself on this continuum?

Very competitive _____ 1
Very competitive, somewhat cooperative _____ 2
Equally competitive and cooperative _____ 3 (40)
Somewhat competitive, very cooperative _____ 4
Very cooperative _____ 5

72. Are you in favor in medical school of a letter grading system, or a Pass-Fail system? (Check one)

Letter Grading System _____ 1 (41)
Pass-Fail _____ 2

CARE IN SCARCITY AREAS

73. Would you be in favor of a National Service Corps for physicians, in which every physician, male or female, would have to serve one or two years in a medically deprived area in order to obtain a permanent license? (Check one)

Yes____1
No____2   (42)

74. Would you work in a medical institution such as a hospital or a clinic, in which the consumers are the majority of the governing board? (Check one)

Yes____1
No____2   (43)

75. Who do you feel should set physicians fees? (Check one)

Physicians____1
Consumer groups____2   (44)
Bargaining between the two groups____3

76. A proposal has been made for a National Insurance Plan in which each person able to pay has a certain amount added to his or her annual income tax; the government pays for those unable to pay; and the government uses these funds to pay for medical care. Are you in favor of such a plan?

Yes____1
No____2   (45)

77. If a National Insurance Plan is passed by Congress, do you think it should: (Check one)

A. Include the total population ____1
B. Include only those too poor to   (46)
   purchase services themselves ____2

78. Should a National Insurance Plan: (Check one)

A. Give funds to the consumer to
   pay for services ____1
B. Regulate the use of funds so
   that the system for the   (47)
   delivery of health care is
   changed ____2

79. Which do you think will be the prevailing mode of medical practice in 1980? (Check one)

Solo practice, fee for service ____1
Group parctice, fee for service ____2
Group practice, monthly pre-payment plan ____3   (48)
All physicians employed by the government ____4

80. Rank order the importance of <u>each</u> of the following supportive programs as an incentive for physicians to practice in a medically deprived area. "1" would indicate that it is of great importance, "4" that it is of little importance

	1	2	3	4
Not having to pay back the loans for medical education.	____	____	____	____
Scholarship for all expenses in medical school.	____	____	____	____
Membership in a group practice.	____	____	____	____
Medical school appointment.	____	____	____	____
Large annual income.	____	____	____	____

(49-53)

81. How much has your career been affected by the following? (check <u>one</u> category on each line)

	1 None	2 Slightly	3 Moderately	4 Greatly
Economic Factors:	____	____	____	____
Social Factors:	____	____	____	____
Other:	____	____	____	____

(54-56)

What?_____

Would you comment on how any of the above factors have been important in your reaching your present career?

_____

_____

_____

82. There is great difficulty in defining "family practice". Do you consider yourself primarily a family practitioner?

Yes____ 1
No____ 2   (57)

If the answer is "Yes", what is the vehicle?   (Check one)

General internal medicine____ 1
General pediatrics____ 2
General practitioner____ 3
Other, what?_____ 4

(58)

Col. (80) - 4

Senior Questionnaire

_____(1-5,6)

NAME_____

MEDICAL SCHOOL_____

TODAY'S DATE_____

YEAR ENTERED MEDICAL SCHOOL (Check One)   Before 1969_____1
                                                  1969_____2
                                                  1970_____3   (8)
                                                  1971_____4
                                                  1972_____5

SEX (Check one)   Male_____1
                                                Female_____2   (9)

AGE   _____   (10-11)

MARITAL STATUS (Check one)   Single_____1
                                                Married_____2
                                               Divorced_____3   (12)
                                              Separated_____4

If you are married, divorced or separated...
                                At what age did you marry?_____   (13-14)

    At what point in your career did you marry? (Check one)

                                   Before college_____1
                         First two years of college_____2
                          Last two years of college_____3   (15)
                     First two years of med school_____4
                      Last two years of med school_____5

CHILDREN? (Check one)   Yes_____1   (16)
                                                     No_____2

PLEASE READ <u>ALL</u> DIRECTIONS CAREFULLY

1. What is your father's occupation? Be specific. (If retired or deceased, record this fact and indicate his former occupation.)

    _____ (17)

2. What is your father's education? (Circle highest level attained)

    GRADE SCHOOL   HIGH SCHOOL   COLLEGE   POST-GRADUATE
    1 2 3 4 5 6 7 8   9 10 11 12   13 14 15 16   17 18 19 20 and over   (18-19)

3. What is your mother's education? (Circle highest level attained)

    GRADE SCHOOL   HIGH SCHOOL   COLLEGE   POST-GRADUATE
    1 2 3 4 5 6 7 8   9 10 11 10   13 14 15 16   17 18 19 20 and over   (20-21)

4. What is your mother's present occupation? Be specific.

    If Housewife, check here____1 _____ _____ (22)

5. Which of the following best describes the place where you grew up? (Check one)

    A farm or ranch_____1
    A town of less than 10,000_____2
    A small city of from 10,000 to 100,000_____3
    A suburb of a large city_____4   (23)
    Within a large city_____5
    You moved so much it would be hard to say_____6

6. Is or was your mother or father a doctor?

    Neither_____1
    Mother_____2
    Father_____3   (24)
    Both_____4

7. Did you ever interrupt your undergraduate college education for a year or more? (Check one)

    Yes_____1
    No_____2   (25)

8. Indicate how many summers you worked in the following areas before medical school:

    Hospital work with patients_____
    Lab assistant or technician in a hospital_____
    Research_____   (26-30)
    Work in slums or rural areas_____
    Other_____
    What?_____

9. How many summers was it necessary for you to earn money to support
    yourself as an undergraduate in college?

none	_____	0	
1	_____	1	
2	_____	2	
3	_____	3	(31)
4	_____	4	

    ... in medical school?

none	_____	0	
1	_____	1	
2	_____	2	
3	_____	3	(32)
4	_____	4	

10. Did you have to work to support yourself during the academic year as
    an undergraduate at college (excluding summers)?

Yes	_____	1	
No	_____	2	(33)

    ... in medical school?

Yes	_____	1	
No	_____	2	(34)

11. From which type of secondary school were you graduated? (Check one)

Public	_____	1	
Private	_____	2	(35)
Parochial	_____	3	

12. <u>Rank</u> the following subjects according to the amount of pleasure they
    gave you during college by writing "1" for the most enjoyable subject,
    <u>and so on</u> to "4" for the least enjoyable subject.

    Rank assigned

Natural sciences	_____
Behavioral sciences	_____
Humanities	_____
Social sciences	_____

13. Did you do any research while an undergraduate at college?

Yes	_____	1	
No	_____	2	(40)

    ... in medical school?

Yes	_____	1	
No	_____	2	(41)

14. If you did any research during college, specify which field: (Check the predominant field)

Biology	1	
Chemistry	2	
Biochemistry	3	
Engineering or Physical Science	4	(42)
Public Health	5	
Social Sciences	6	
Behavioral Sciences	7	
Other	8	
What?		

...in medical school:

Basic Sciences	1	
Clinical Sciences	2	
Psychiatry	3	(43)
Public Health	4	
Other (specify)	5	

15. If you had not been going to medical school, would you have preferred to major in something else while in college? (Check one)

Yes	1	(44)
No	2	

If the answer is <u>yes</u>, would it have been:
(Check one)

A Science	1	
Humanities	2	
Social Science	3	(45)
Psychology	4	
Don't Know	5	
Other - What?	6	

If the answer is yes, did you elect your college major because: (Check one)

A The curriculum in my college was so set up that this major allowed me to take the electives that I wanted _____ 1

B. I thought it the best way to get into medical school _____ 2 (46)

C. I thought it the best way to prepare for medical school _____ 3

D. I made an understandable mistake _____ 4

E. It was the subject I was most interested in _____ 5

16. Before deciding on medicine, did you ever seriously consider any other occupation or profession? (Check one)

Yes_____1
No_____2

(47)

If yes, did you ever seriously consider a career in one or more of the following fields? (Check as many as apply)

Sciences, PhD level_____
Humanities, PhD level_____
Social Sciences, PhD level_____
Psychology, PhD level_____
Becoming a businessman or woman_____
Becoming a lawyer_____
Becoming a teacher of elementary
or secondary school_____
Becoming a Social Worker_____
Going to a School of Public Health_____
Becoming a Hospital Administrator_____
Becoming an Engineer_____
Becoming an Architect_____
Other, What?_____

(48-60)

17. Did you have difficulty in making up your mind whether to pursue an M.D. or PhD?

Yes_____1
No_____2

(61)

If yes, which of the following areas did you consider for a PhD? (Check one)

Natural Sciences_____1
Behavioral Sciences_____2
Humanities_____3
Social Sciences_____4

(62)

18. If on several attempts, you had failed to secure entrance to any medical
     school would you have: (Check one)

                Gone to graduate schools in the natural
                                     sciences_____1
                Gone to graduate school in the humanities_____2
                Gone to graduate school in the social
                                     sciences_____3
                Gone to graduate school in psychology_____4
                          Become a businessman_____5
                            Become a Lawyer_____6
                Become a teacher of elementary or
                          secondary school_____7   (63-64)
                       Gone to Dental School_____8
                   Gone to Social Work School_____9
                Gone to a School of Public Health_____10
                Become a Hospital Administrator_____11
                Become an Engineer or Architect_____12
                             Other, What?_____13

19. When did you <u>first</u> think of becoming a physician? (Check one)

                            Before college_____1
                    First two years of college_____2
                              Junior year_____3   (65)
                              Senior year_____4
                            After college_____5

20. When did you <u>consolidate</u> your career plans to become a physician?
     (Check one)

                            Before college_____1
                    First two years of college_____2
                              Junior year_____3   (66)
                              Senior year_____4
                            After college_____5

21. <u>Rank</u> the following subjects according to the grades you received in them
     in college by writing "1" for the highest grades, "2" for the next, and
     so on to "4".

                                        Rank assigned

                        Natural sciences_____
                     Behavioral sciences_____   (67-70)
                             Humanities_____
                        Social sciences_____

22. What was your college major or field of concentration? (Check one)

Biochemical Sciences_____1
Biochemistry_____2
Biology_____3
Biophysics_____4
Chemistry_____5
Cultural Anthropology_____6
Economics_____7   (71-72)
Engineering_____8
Government or Political Science_____9
Humanities_____10
Mathematics_____11
Physics_____12
Pre-Med_____13
Psychology_____14
Sociology_____15

23. When you entered college did you plan to: (Check one)

Become a physician_____1
Go to graduate school in the sciences_____2
Go to graduate school in the humanities_____3
Go to graduate school in the social
sciences_____4
Go to graduate school in psychology_____5
Become a businessman_____6
Become a lawyer_____7
Become a teacher of elementary or   (73-74)
secondary school_____8
Go to dental school_____9
Go to social work school_____10
Go to a school of public health_____11
Become a hospital administrator_____12
Become an engineer or architect_____13
Undecided_____14
Other, What?_____15

Col. 80-1

CAREER CHOICE

The following vignettes are descriptions of various careers of physicians. Please read them carefully since you will be asked to answer questions about the one which best corresponds to your present career.

CAREER NUMBER 1

This physician is a clinical <u>Subspecialist</u>. This doctor's education is basic-ally bioscientific. If an internist, he or she is a cardiologist, gastro-enterologist, allergist, etc. If a surgeon, an orthopedic surgeon, plastic surgeon, abdominal surgeon, neurosurgeon, etc. If in pediatrics, a pediatric cardiologist, a pediatric allergist, etc. If not in a subspecialty of a major specialty, he or she is in a specialty whose scope is narrowly defined. Examples of this would be neurology, pathology, radiology, etc.

CAREER NUMBER 2

This physician is a <u>General Specialist</u>. This doctor's education is basically bioscientific, but he or she is more interested in a broad range of problems within a specialty rather than a subspecialty. Examples of this are general internal medicine, general pediatrics, general surgery, etc.

CAREER NUMBER 3

This physician is a <u>Basic Scientist.</u> This doctor has no clinical practice, but is totally engaged in teaching and research in a basic science.

CAREER NUMBER 4

This physician is a <u>Biomedical Engineer</u>. This doctor majored in college in a physical science such as mathematics, computer science, engineering or physics and has a career dealing with medical problems which involve his or her knowledge of these sciences.

CAREER NUMBER 5

This physician is a <u>Psychiatrist</u>, primarily concerned with patients with psychological problems or mental illnesses.

CAREER NUMBER 6

This physician is a <u>Public Health Physician</u>. He or she not only has a medical education, but possibly also a degree in public health. This doctor deals directly with preventing diseases, research into their prevention, or into the problems of health care delivery, or administers either a hospital or community clinic.

CAREER NUMBER 7

This physician is a General Practitioner with the new name of <u>Family Practitioner</u>. He or she is engaged in diagnosis and treating not only patients' physical problems, but also the related family, social, and emotional aspects of the patients' illness. He or she has a broad training in internal medicine, pediatrics, minor surgery, and obstetrics and gynecology, and closely resembles the old style general practitioner.

24. Although none of these careers would exactly correspond to your plans, which
     one most nearly corresponds to the 1st choice career you <u>plan</u> to follow?

                    <u>First</u> choice career number _____

              Which career would be your <u>second</u> choice? _____   (6-8)

           Which career would you <u>least</u> like to pursue? _____

25. How certain are you that you will follow through on this <u>planned</u>
     career? (Check one)

                              Very certain _____ 1

                                  Certain _____ 2   (9)

                                 Doubtful _____ 3

26. Is there a career which you prefer to the one you ranked as your
     Number 1 planned career in question 24? (Check one)

                                     Yes _____ 1

                                      No _____ 2   (10)

27. Rank the following factors in order of their importance in the choice of
     your career by writing "1" for the most important, "2" for the next in
     importance, and so on. If any one or more of these factors are not
     important, omit them from the ranking.

                                                 Rank assigned

          Intellectual content of the career   _____
          Example of a physician in this career   _____
          Social factors, such as colleagues,
             type of patient, etc.   _____   (11-15)
          Working hours   _____
          Other   _____
             What?_____

SPECIALTY CHOICE

28.   Check your planned specialty:

<table>
<tr><td>Medicine, general</td><td>_____</td><td>1</td></tr>
<tr><td>Medicine, subspecialty</td><td></td><td></td></tr>
<tr><td>   Allergy and immunology</td><td>_____</td><td>2</td></tr>
<tr><td>   Cardiology</td><td>_____</td><td>3</td></tr>
<tr><td>   Gastroenterology</td><td>_____</td><td>4</td></tr>
<tr><td>   Pulmonary diseases</td><td>_____</td><td>5</td></tr>
<tr><td>   Other medical sub-</td><td></td><td></td></tr>
<tr><td>   specialty, what?_____</td><td></td><td>6</td></tr>
<tr><td>Surgery, general</td><td>_____</td><td>7</td></tr>
<tr><td>Surgery, subspecialty</td><td></td><td></td></tr>
<tr><td>   Abdominal</td><td>_____</td><td>8</td></tr>
<tr><td>   Neurosurgery</td><td>_____</td><td></td></tr>
<tr><td>   Orthopedic surgery</td><td>_____</td><td>10</td></tr>
<tr><td>   Plastic surgery</td><td>_____</td><td>11</td></tr>
<tr><td>   Thoracic surgery</td><td>_____</td><td>12</td></tr>
<tr><td>   Urology</td><td>_____</td><td>13</td></tr>
<tr><td>   Other surgical sub-</td><td></td><td></td></tr>
<tr><td>   specialty, what?_____</td><td></td><td>14</td></tr>
<tr><td>Other specialties</td><td></td><td></td></tr>
<tr><td>   Anesthesiology</td><td>_____</td><td>15</td></tr>
<tr><td>   Basic scientist</td><td>_____</td><td>16</td></tr>
<tr><td>   Dermatology</td><td>_____</td><td>17</td></tr>
<tr><td>   Family (General</td><td></td><td>(16-17)</td></tr>
<tr><td>   practice)</td><td>_____</td><td>18</td></tr>
<tr><td>   Nuclear medicine</td><td>_____</td><td>19</td></tr>
<tr><td>   Obstetrics and</td><td></td><td></td></tr>
<tr><td>   gynecology</td><td>_____</td><td>20</td></tr>
<tr><td>   Ophthalmology</td><td>_____</td><td>21</td></tr>
<tr><td>   Otolaryngology</td><td>_____</td><td>22</td></tr>
<tr><td>   Pathology</td><td>_____</td><td>23</td></tr>
<tr><td>   Pediatrics (General)</td><td>_____</td><td>24</td></tr>
<tr><td>   Pediatrics subspecialty</td><td></td><td></td></tr>
<tr><td>   Allergist</td><td>_____</td><td>25</td></tr>
<tr><td>   Cardiologist</td><td>_____</td><td>26</td></tr>
<tr><td>   Physical medicine and</td><td></td><td></td></tr>
<tr><td>   rehabilitation</td><td>_____</td><td>27</td></tr>
<tr><td>   Public Health:</td><td></td><td></td></tr>
<tr><td>   Bacterial</td><td>_____</td><td>28</td></tr>
<tr><td>   Environmental</td><td>_____</td><td>29</td></tr>
<tr><td>   Health care delivery</td><td>_____</td><td>30</td></tr>
<tr><td>   Psychiatry</td><td>_____</td><td>31</td></tr>
<tr><td>   Neurology</td><td>_____</td><td>32</td></tr>
<tr><td>   Radiology</td><td>_____</td><td>33</td></tr>
<tr><td>   Other - What?_____</td><td></td><td>34</td></tr>
</table>

MODE OF WORK

29. Even though you may not have arrived at a definite choice for your planned mode of work, place a "1" next to your first choice, and a "2" next to your second choice (DO NOT RANK ALL ITEMS - RANK ONLY 2 ITEMS)

Full time medical school faculty	_____	1
Part time medical school faculty; part time private practice solo, or part time practice group	_____	2
Full time private practice solo or group, with no medical school affiliation	_____	3
Full time government employee	_____	4
Part time government employee; part time medical school	_____	5	(18-20)
Part time government employee; part time private practice, solo or group	_____	6
Don't know	_____	7
Other - what?	_____	8

_____

IN THE ABOVE LIST, PLACE AN "X" NEXT TO THE MODE OF WORK YOU WOULD LEAST LIKE TO FOLLOW.

30. In your career, where do you plan to derive <u>MOST</u> of your <u>INCOME</u>?
    (Check one)

Solo practice, fee for service	_____	1
Group practice fee for service	_____	2
Group practice, monthly prepaid	_____	3
Medical school employment	_____	4
Hospital employment	_____	5
Government employment	_____	6

(21)

31. How do you expect to obtain most of your patients? (Check one)

Referred by other doctors	_____	1
By being selected by the patient	_____	2
Assigned by rotation in a group or hospital practice	_____	3

(22)

PLACE OF WORK

32. It is now possible, whether you are in private practice or academic
    medicine, to choose the location of your work with patients. <u>Rank</u>
    order <u>all</u> of the following in order of your preference, from "1" --
    most preferred -- to "7" -- least preferred.

	Rank assigned
Ghetto	_____
Rural	_____
Suburban	_____
Urban-non-ghetto	_____
Foreign country	_____
Indian reservation	_____
Military service	_____

(23-29)

33. Are there any discrepancies between the location you would <u>LIKE</u> to work
    and the location you <u>EXPECT</u> to work? (Check one)

Yes	_____	1
No	_____	2

(30)

If the answer is <u>yes</u>, please explain the discrepancies._____

_____

_____

34. What percentage of your time do you plan to work in the following
    areas? (Amounts should total 100%)

	Percent	
Ghetto	_____	(31-33)
Rural	_____	(34-36)
Suburban	_____	(37-39)
Urban, no-ghetto	_____	(40-42)
Foreign country	_____	(43-45)
Indian Reservation	_____	(46-48)
Military service	_____	(49-51)
Total	100%	

TIME ALLOTMENT

35. As a physician, approximately what percentage of time would you ideally
    <u>LIKE</u> to spend in each of the following professional activities?
    (Amounts should total 100%)

	Percent	
Research	_____	(52-54)
Taking care of patients	_____	(55-57)
Administration	_____	(58-60)
Teaching	_____	(61-63)
Total	100%	

36. Approximately what percentage of your time do you <u>EXPECT</u> to spend in the following activities? (Amounts should total 100%)

	Percent	
Research	_____	(64-66)
Taking care of patients	_____	(67-69)
Administration	_____	(70-72)
Teaching	_____	(73-75)
Total	100%	

37. Are there any discrepancies between how you would <u>LIKE</u> to spend your time and how you <u>EXPECT</u> to spend your time? (Check one)

Yes _____ 1

No _____ 2

(76)

If the answer is <u>yes</u>, please explain the discrepancies:_____

_____

_____

Col. 80-2

38. Of the time that you <u>EXPECT</u> to spend in taking care of patients, approximately what percentage of this time would be devoted to the following: (Amounts should total 100%)

	Percent	
Hospitalized patients	_____	(6-8)
Ambulatory care of patients previously hospitalized	_____	(9-11)
Office care of patients, not hospitalized but requiring the care of a specialist	_____	(12-14)
Primary care, day-to-day care of illnesses which could also be treated by a family (general) practitioner i.e. first patient contact practice	_____	(15-17)
Total	100%	

39. In your career, where do you plan to spend <u>MOST</u> of your <u>TIME</u>?
    (Check one)

Solo practice, fee for service	_____	1
Group practice, fee for service	_____	2
Group practice, monthly prepaid	_____	3
Medical school faculty	_____	4
Hospital employment	_____	5
Government employment	_____	6

(18)

40. Twenty years from now, how many hours per week...

Do you <u>EXPECT</u> to work professionally? (Check one)

20-30 hrs.	_____	1
31-40 hrs.	_____	2
41-50 hrs.	_____	3
51-60 hrs.	_____	4
Over 61 hrs.	_____	5

(19)

Would you <u>LIKE</u> to work professionally? (Check one)

20-30 hrs.	_____	1
31-40 hrs.	_____	2
41-50 hrs.	_____	3
51-60 hrs.	_____	4
Over 61 hrs.	_____	5

(20)

41. If there is a discrepancy between the number of hours you expect to
    work professionally and the number you would like to work, do you feel
    that this will be because of: (Check as many as you feel appropriate)

    a. Family needs _____ (21)

    b. Availability of opportunities to
       do what you would like to do out-
       side of medicine _____ (22)

    c. Pressure from demands of practice _____ (23)

    d. Competitive pressures derived from
       wish for advancement _____ (24)

    e. Other _____ (25)

       What? _____

       _____

GENERAL

42. Which phase of your medical training do you think will be the most important for your later career in medicine? (Check one)

<table>
<tr><td>First two years of medical school</td><td>_____</td><td>1</td><td></td></tr>
<tr><td>Last two years of medical school</td><td>_____</td><td>2</td><td></td></tr>
<tr><td>Internship</td><td>_____</td><td>3</td><td>(26)</td></tr>
<tr><td>Residency</td><td>_____</td><td>4</td><td></td></tr>
<tr><td>Don't know</td><td>_____</td><td>5</td><td></td></tr>
</table>

43. At the present time, do you have any doubts about medicine as a career for you? (Check one)

<table>
<tr><td>Yes, serious doubts</td><td>_____</td><td>1</td><td></td></tr>
<tr><td>Yes, slight doubts</td><td>_____</td><td>2</td><td></td></tr>
<tr><td>A few doubts</td><td>_____</td><td>3</td><td>(27)</td></tr>
<tr><td>No doubts at all</td><td>_____</td><td>4</td><td></td></tr>
</table>

44. Have you had doubts about whether you wished an M.D or a PhD? (Check one)

<table>
<tr><td>Yes, serious doubts</td><td>_____</td><td>1</td><td></td></tr>
<tr><td>Yes, slight doubts</td><td>_____</td><td>2</td><td></td></tr>
<tr><td>A few doubts</td><td>_____</td><td>3</td><td>(28)</td></tr>
<tr><td>No doubts at all</td><td>_____</td><td>4</td><td></td></tr>
</table>

45. Do you NOW have doubts about whether you wish an M.D. or a PhD? (Check one)

<table>
<tr><td>Yes, serious doubts</td><td>_____</td><td>1</td><td></td></tr>
<tr><td>Yes, slight doubts</td><td>_____</td><td>2</td><td></td></tr>
<tr><td>A few doubts</td><td>_____</td><td>3</td><td>(29)</td></tr>
<tr><td>No doubts at all</td><td>_____</td><td>4</td><td></td></tr>
</table>

46. Have you or do you plan to get a Phd? (Check one)

<table>
<tr><td>Yes</td><td>_____</td><td>1</td><td>(30)</td></tr>
<tr><td>No</td><td>_____</td><td>2</td><td></td></tr>
</table>

47. On which activities are you interested in spending time <u>after</u> graduation from medical school? <u>Rank</u> them in order of their importance by writing "1" for the most important, "2" for the next in importance, <u>and so on for each activity on the list</u>. (Rank <u>all</u> 6 items.)

<u>Rank assigned</u>

Career or occupation	_____	(31)
Leisure-time recreational activities	_____	(32)
Participation as citizen in affairs of own community	_____	(33)
Family relationships	_____	(34)
Religious beliefs or activities	_____	(35)
Activities directed toward national or international betterment	_____	(36)

48. After you have completed your residency training, which of the following will be your means of keeping up with advances in medicine? (Express your answer in terms of a <u>percentage</u>, including the "Other - What?" category if it applies: (Amounts should total 100%)

	<u>Percent</u>	
Reading journals and books	_____%	(37-39)
Attending medical meetings	_____%	(40-42)
Taking post-graduate course	_____%	(43-45)
Hospital rounds	_____%	(46-48)
Other - What? _____	_____%	(49-51)

_____

_____

49. <u>Rank</u> the following men in order from the person most admired, "1", to the person least admired, "3".

	Rank	
Churchill	_____	(52)
Pasteur	_____	(53)
Freud	_____	(54)

50. What are your reactions -- negative, neutral or positive -- to the following types of patients? (Check <u>one</u> for <u>each</u> type of patient)

	<u>Negative</u>	<u>Neutral</u>	<u>Positive</u>	
Children	___ 1	___ 2	___ 3	(55)
Young people	___ 1	___ 2	___ 3	(56)
People with terminal illnesses	___ 1	___ 2	___ 3	(57)
People who have psychogenic symptoms	___ 1	___ 2	___ 3	(58)
Old people	___ 1	___ 2	___ 3	(59)
People who have clearcut physical illnesses	___ 1	___ 2	___ 3	(60)
Poor people	___ 1	___ 2	___ 3	(61)
Rich people	___ 1	___ 2	___ 3	(62)
The worried well	___ 1	___ 2	___ 3	(63)

FINANCING YOUR MEDICAL EDUCATION

51. How difficult was it for you to finance your medical education? (Check one)

Very difficult	___ 1	
Fairly difficult	___ 2	
Not very difficult	___ 3	(64)
Not at all difficult	___ 4	

Col. 80-3

52. What percentage of your medical education expenses did you receive
    from the following sources? (The amounts should total 100%.)

Parents _____	%	(6-8)
Spouse _____	%	(9-11)
Other relatives _____	%	(12-14)
Scholarship _____	%	(15-17)
Loans _____	%	(18-20)
Personal Earnings _____	%	(21-23)
GI Bill of Rights _____	%	(24-26)
Armed Services or Public Health Services _____	%	(27-29)

Total 100%

53. Have you received any scholarship aid for your medical education?
    (Check one)

Yes _____ 1

No _____ 2   (30)

54. Do you owe money for your medical education? (Check one)

Yes _____ 1

No _____ 2   (31)

If YES, approximately how much do you owe? (Check one)

Less than $1000 _____ 1
$1000-$2000 _____ 2
$2000-$5000 _____ 3
$5000-$10000 _____ 4   (32)
$10000-$15000 _____ 5
More than $15000 _____ 6

55. What things do you think you will like best about being a doctor? (Check
     <u>one</u> category on each line)

	Like to a very great extent	Like to a great extent	Like to some extent	Like to a little extent	Like to a very little extent	
Being able to deal directly with people	1	2	3	4	5	(33)
Being able to help other people	1	2	3	4	5	(34)
The fact that medicine is a highly respected profession	1	2	3	4	5	(35)
Having interesting and intelligent people for colleagues	1	2	3	4	5	(36)
Doing work involving scientific method	1	2	3	4	5	(37)
Being my own boss	1	2	3	4	5	(38)
Being sure of earning an excellent income	1	2	3	4	5	(39)
The challenging and stimulating nature of the work	1	2	3	4	5	(40)
Using medicine to change society or the social system	1	2	3	4	5	(41)
Dealing with the psychological problems of patients	1	2	3	4	5	(42)
Ability to combine working with people with research	1	2	3	4	5	(43)
The fact that, within medicine, if certain career patterns are followed an individual can attain great prestige and status	1	2	3	4	5	(44)

56. A physician can be of service to his patients in a number of ways. Rank order the importance you attach to the following with a "1" for "most important" to a "3" for "least important." Rank all three items on the list.

                                          Rank Assigned

                 Doing research on the
                 problems of disease   _____   (45)

                 Treating patients
                 directly   _____   (46)

                 Preventive medicine   _____   (47)

57. Do you plan to be politically active with respect to questions of health on the community and/or national level? (Check one)

                                          Yes _____ 1
                                          No _____ 2   (48)

58. In the running of a Neighborhood Clinic, which of the following administrative arrangements do you prefer? Policy is decided by: (Check one)

                 Representatives of the community;
                 the physicians carry them out   _____ 1

                 The community and the physicians
                 on an equal basis   _____ 2   (49)

                 The physicians, after consultation
                 with the community   _____ 3

59. In securing changes in the delivery of medical care to the community, which do you favor? (Check one)

                 Action without careful analysis and
                 research, but evaluation afterwards
                 making changes as necessary   _____ 1

                 Careful analysis and research before   (50)
                 action   _____ 2

60. Do you plan to be politically active in other social issues on the community and/or national level? (Check one)

                                          Yes _____ 1
                                          No _____ 2   (51)

61. Do you think "fee for service" should be retained for the majority of physicians? (Check one)

Yes _____ 1
No _____ 2   (52)

For yourself? (Check one)

Yes _____ 1
No _____ 2   (53)

62. Do you think the majority of physicians should be in group practice or solo practice? (Check one)

Group _____ 1
Solo _____ 2   (54)

Which do you prefer for yourself? (Check one)

Group _____ 1
Solo _____ 2   (55)

If you prefer a group practice for yourself, do you favor a multi-specialist group or a uni-specialist group? (Check one)

Multi-specialist _____ 1
Uni-specialist _____ 2   (56)

63. If you prefer a group practice, how important are each of the following for your choice of group practice? Give each a percentage with all totaling 100%.

A group would enable me to control my hours of work, so that the increased efficiency, coupled with much less night work, would allow me to spend more time with my family and on other activities outside of medicine. _____% (57-59)

Increase the level of competency of the practice of medicine, since a group of physicians with varied training can give a higher level of care, than one physician who does all things. _____% (60-62)

The pooling of office expenses thus lowering the costs of practice and making possible laboratory and x-ray facilities as well as allied health personnel, which would not be possible in solo practice. _____% (63-65)

Total: 100%

64. For your internship, which type of hospital would you choose: (Check one)

    A. Highly specialized hospital   _____ 1

    B. Out-patient Community

        Oriented Hospital   _____ 2 (66)

65. Ten years from now, when you are launched in your career, which type of hospital would you prefer to be affiliated with: (Check one)

    A. Highly specialized hospital   _____ 1

    B. Out-patient Community

        Oriented Hospital   _____ 2 (67)

66. Would you like to work on a full-time basis for the government? (Check one)

        Yes _____ 1 (68)

        No _____ 2

67. In your practice would you utilize the following assistants? (Check any you would use)

    High school graduate with two years

    specialized training   _____ (69)

    Nurse with additional two years

    training   _____ (70)

    College graduate with a Baccalaureate

    Degree educated as a doctor's assistant   _____ (71)

    Two-Year Junior College graduate trained

    as a doctor's assistant   _____ (72)

    Discharged Navy Corpsmen   _____ (73)

68. Would you utilize paramedical personnel in the following areas? (Check the areas if you would utilize the personnel)

    Minor surgery   _____ (74)

    Well-baby clinic   _____ (75)

    Handling emotional, social and family

    aspects of patients with physical

    problems   _____ (76)

    Diagnosis and treatment of minor

    illnesses   _____ (77)

Col. 80-4

69. <u>Rank</u> order the importance to you of the following areas of social responsibility by writing "1" for the most important, "2" for the next in importance, <u>and so on for each statement</u>. Rank <u>all five</u> statements.

Rank Assigned

Attention to the emotional, social, and family aspects of the care of patients; i.e., The Art of Medicine   _____   (6)

Technological and scientific competence of a physician   _____   (7)

Delivery of optimal care to all segments of the population without regard to finances   _____   (8)

Research   _____   (9)

A Preventive Medicine which takes action on the social factors which cause disease and which impedes health   _____   (10)

70. In his concern with the social factors, such as housing, education, hunger, etc., which impede health and produce disease, should the physician's prime effort be: (Check the <u>one</u> most important to you)

To change these factors through political action with the community   _____ 1

To develop with the community, neighborhood clinics and Public Health programs aimed at finding people who are ill and making modern care available to them   _____ 2   (11)

The physician should not be concerned with social factors   _____ 3

71. Have the cuts in research funds affected your career choice? (Check one)

Yes _____ 1   (12)
No _____ 2

If the answer is "Yes", in what way? _____

_____

_____

_____

72. Are you in favor of the states requiring each physician to take an examination for relicensure every six years? (Check one)

Yes _____	1
No _____	2 (13)

73. Which of the following do you esteem most highly? <u>Rank</u> them from the highest "1", to the lowest "3". Rank <u>all three</u> items.

Rank Assigned

Intellectual tasks	_____	(14)
Interpersonal relationships	_____	(15)
Introspection	_____	(16)

74. Were you on a varsity athletic team in college? (Check one)

Yes _____	1 (17)
No _____	2

75. Regardless of whether you were on a varsity team, rate your athletic ability (Check one)

Excellent	_____	1
Good	_____	2 (18)
Fair	_____	3
Poor	_____	4

76. Do you like to work with your hands? (Check one)

Very much	_____	1
Some	_____	2 (19)
Little	_____	3

77. How skillful are you in doing mechanical work? (Check one)

Excellent	_____	1
Good	_____	2 (20)
Fair	_____	3
Poor	_____	4

78. Which of the following most accurately describes the type of physician
you wish to become? (Check one)

> Primarily a scientist, who helps people
> by treating their illnesses using a
> high level of scientific knowledge _____ 1
>
> Primarily interested in working directly
> with people, being of service to them,
> treating their illnesses using science   (21)
> pragmatically _____ 2

79. Many have stated that for high scientific achievement, competition must
be stimulated in order that the most able students academically emerge
to do science and secure the research grants. On the other hand, it is
stated that the delivery of medical care requires the development of
cooperative physicians who can work well with other physicians, health
workers, patients and communities. These two views of physicians are
the antithesis of each other. They can be placed at the two ends of a
continuum as competitive versus cooperative. Where would you place yourself on this continuum?

> Very competitive _____ 1
> Very competitive, somewhat cooperative _____ 2
> Equally competitive and cooperative _____ 3 (22)
> Somewhat competitive, very cooperative _____ 4
> Very cooperative _____ 5

80. How much do you expect to earn, twenty years from now, keeping the value
of the dollar constant, i.e., at today's prices:

> Less than $20,000 _____ 1
> 20,000 to 30,000 _____ 2
> 30,000 to 40,000 _____ 3 (23)
> 40,000 to 50,000 _____ 4
> 50,000 to 75,000 _____ 5
> more than 75,000 _____ 6

81. Are you in favor in medical school of a letter or numerical grading
system, or a Pass-Fail system? (Check one)

> Letter or numerical
> Grading System _____ 1
> Pass-Fail _____ 2 (24)

CARE IN SCARCITY AREAS

82. Would you be in favor of a National Service Corps for physicians, in which every physician, male or female, would have to serve one or two years in a medically deprived area in order to obtain a permanent license? (Check one)

$$\begin{array}{ll} \text{Yes} \underline{\hspace{1cm}} & 1 \\ \text{No} \underline{\hspace{1cm}} & 2 \end{array} \quad (25)$$

83. Would you work in a medical institution such as a hospital or a clinic, in which the consumers are the majority of the governing board? (Check one)

$$\begin{array}{ll} \text{Yes} \underline{\hspace{1cm}} & 1 \\ \text{No} \underline{\hspace{1cm}} & 2 \end{array} \quad (26)$$

84. Who do you feel should set physicians fees? (Check one)

$$\begin{array}{ll} \text{Physicians} \underline{\hspace{1cm}} & 1 \\ \text{Consumer groups} \underline{\hspace{1cm}} & 2 \\ \text{Bargaining between the two groups} \underline{\hspace{1cm}} & 3 \end{array} \quad (27)$$

85. A proposal has been made for a National Health Insurance Plan in which each person able to pay has a certain amount added to his annual income tax; the government pays for those unable to pay; and the government uses these funds to pay for medical care. Are you in favor of such a plan?

$$\begin{array}{ll} \text{Yes} \underline{\hspace{1cm}} & 1 \\ \text{No} \underline{\hspace{1cm}} & 2 \end{array} \quad (28)$$

86. If a National Health Insurance Plan is passed by Congress, do you think it should: (Check one)

$$\begin{array}{ll} \text{Include the total population?} & \underline{\hspace{1cm}} \ 1 \\ \text{Include only those too poor to purchase} & \\ \text{services themselves?} & \underline{\hspace{1cm}} \ 2 \end{array} \quad (29)$$

87. Should a National Health Insurance Plan: (Check one)

$$\begin{array}{ll} \text{Give funds to the consumer to pay} & \\ \text{services?} & \underline{\hspace{1cm}} \ 1 \\ \text{Regulate the use of funds so that the} & \\ \text{system for the delivery of health} & \\ \text{care is changed?} & \underline{\hspace{1cm}} \ 2 \end{array} \quad (30)$$

88. Which do you think will be the prevailing mode of medical practice in 1985? (Check one)

Solo practice, fee for service	_____	1
Group practice, fee for service	_____	2
Group practice, monthly pre-payment plan	_____	3 (31)
All physicians employed by the government	_____	4

89. Check one of the following:

1. I plan to practice in a medically deprived area regardless of any supportive programs _____ 1

2. No combination of supportive programs would convince me to practice in a medically deprived area. _____ 2 (32)

3. I would practice in a medically deprived area if certain supportive programs were available _____ 3

90. If you checked 3 in the above question, indicate the importance of <u>each</u> of the following supportive programs, as an incentive for <u>you</u> to practice in a medically deprived area. (1) would indicate it is of great importance to you, (4) that it is of little importance to you. (Check one category on each line.)

	1	2	3	4	
Not having to pay back the loans for my medical education.	_____	_____	_____	_____	(33)
Scholarship for all expenses in medical school.	_____	_____	_____	_____	(34)
Membership in a group practice.	_____	_____	_____	_____	(35)
Medical school appointment.	_____	_____	_____	_____	(36)
Large annual income.	_____	_____	_____	_____	(37)

91. Indicate the importance of <u>each</u> of the following supportive programs as an incentive for all physicians, not necessarily you, to practice in a medically deprived area. "1" would indicate that it is of great importance, "4" that it is of little importance. (Check one category on each line.)

	1	2	3	4	
Not having to pay back the loans for medical education.	___	___	___	___	(38)
Scholarship for all expenses in medical school.	___	___	___	___	(39)
Membership in a group practice.	___	___	___	___	(40)
Medical school appointment.	___	___	___	___	(41)
Large annual income.	___	___	___	___	(42)

92. How much will your career be affected by the following? (Check <u>one</u> category on each line.)

	1 None	2 Slightly	3 Moderately	4 Greatly	
Economic Factors:	___	___	___	___	(43)
Social Factors:	___	___	___	___	(44)
Other:	___	___	___	___	(45)

What?_____

93. There is great difficulty in defining "family practice". Do you consider that you will be primarily a family practitioner?

Yes _____ 1
No _____ 2   (46)

If the answer is "Yes", what will be the vehicle? (Check one)

General internal medicine _____ 1
General pediatrics _____ 2
General practice _____ 3   (47)
Other, what? _____ 4

94. In which direction do you think medical school admissions policies should
     be changed? To admit ...   (Check one)

                            More scientifically oriented students _____1

                               More people oriented students _____ 2   (48)

95. Rank order the priorities that medical school admission policy should
     give to admitting more of the following students. "1" would indicate
     the highest priority, "3" the lowest.

                                   Rank assigned
                         Scientifically oriented _____   (49)
                         Interpersonally oriented _____   (50)
                         Psychologically oriented _____   (51)

96. Do you consider yourself primarily: (Check one)

                         Scientifically oriented _____ 1
                         Interpersonally oriented _____ 2   (52)
                         Psychologically oriented _____ 3

97. Do you think that medical schools should have two curricula: a
     bioscientific one for the eduction of academicians and sub-
     specialists, the other a biosocial one for the eduction of family
     practitioners, public health physicians, and psychiatrists?
     (Check one)

                                        Yes _____ 1
                                        No _____ 2   (53)

98. Many think that a primary issue in medicine is the depersonalization
     and dehumanization of patient care. Do you agree? (Check one)

                                        Yes _____ 1
                                        No _____ 2   (54)

If your answer is YES, how would you change this? _____

_____

_____

99. How much of a part should other professional medical people such as
Hospital Administrators, Nurses, Social Workers, etc., have in the
decisions relating to medical care delivery? (Check one)

Less than physicians _____ 1

Equal to physicians _____ 2   (55)

More than physicians _____ 3

100. How much of a part should these other professional medical people have
in the decisions concerning individual patient care? (Check one).

Less than the physician _____ 1

Equal to the physician _____ 2   (56)

More than the physician _____ 3

101. Should a National Health Insurance Plan allow for enrollment on a:
(Check one)

Voluntary basis_____ 1

Compulsory basis_____ 2   (57)

102. Are you a transfer student from another medical school? (Check one)

Yes_____ 1

No_____ 2   (58)

If yes, from what school?_____

103. Name the colleges where you received your Pre Medical
Education?

_____   (59)

Col. 80-5

Index

About the Author

Daniel H. Funkenstein is Professor of Psychiatry, Emeritus, Consultant on Admissions to the Dean of the Faculty of Medicine at the Harvard Medical School, and Associate Chief of Staff for Education at the Brockton Veterans Administration Hospital. He has spent more than twenty-five years in research on college and medical students and has published over 100 articles in the field. Long and closely involved in medical school admissions, he has served on a number of national committees concerned with this problem and on national commissions on medical manpower. He has been a visiting professor or lecturer at over fifty medical schools in this country and abroad. For many years, he was chairman of the committee on academic education of the American Psychiatric Association. He also served on numerous committees of the Association of American Medical Colleges.

DATE DUE